manual

Improving Children's Communication

Managing Persistent Communication Difficulties

Poppy Nash, & Louise Toombs

WHURR PUBLISHERS
London & Philadelphia

Improving Children's Communication

Managing Persistent Communication Difficulties

Poppy Nash PhD, MRCSLT
University of York

Jackie Stengelhofen MEd, FRCSLT,
University of Sheffield

Jane Brown MRCSLT **and Louise Toombs** MRCSLT
Swindon Primary Care Trust

Illustrations by David Morris

W
WHURR PUBLISHERS
LONDON AND PHILADELPHIA

British Library Cataloguing in Publication Data

A catalogue record for this book is available from the
British Library.

ISBN 186156 298 5

Printed and bound in the UK by Hobbs the Printers Ltd,
Southampton, Hampshire.

Contents

Foreword

Effective communication is an essential life skill; necessary not only to maintain employment and independence, but also to make friends, form lasting relationships and develop a general feeling of well-being. Thus, it is not surprising that follow-up studies of children with persisting speech and language difficulties have found them to be at risk for associated psychosocial and educational difficulties in later life. Traditionally, intervention for such children has focussed on the younger child's articulation, phonological processes and linguistic structures. Generally, it has been carried out on an individual rather than group basis. Many children make progress through this intervention but not all completely resolve their difficulties – how can we help them?

The intervention programme developed by Nash, Stengelhofen, Brown and Toombs addresses this question. It moves us on from a medical model approach to children's speech and language difficulties to a total management approach in which older children can flourish and take responsibility for their own communication development. It does not abandon the need for an individually tailored programme based on an assessment of strengths and weaknesses and time is given to specific speech work where necessary. However, it is the group context that is used to facilitate communication, share anxieties and good practice, and have fun!

It is an innovative programme in many ways. Perhaps the most obvious is the intensive and residential nature of the course; living together for a short while is an important part of the trust-building on which this programme is based. Sensitive issues such as how to develop conversation, manage the listener, make friends and cope with bullying are addressed through practical activities and the time taken for 'prouding', to reflect on what has been good during the day (i.e. what are you most 'proud' of) is a worthwhile exercise for us all!

What I really like about this publication is the combination of research and practice and how the experience of the authors in these areas shines through. They explain the background to this approach and the rationale for its design. The focus on identifying a Victimise, Ostracise and Stigmatise (VOS) cycle of disadvantage is relevant to all children, as is the objective of strengthening resilience and self-esteem. The authors also provide detailed information about how the courses have been run. Timetables are included as well as specific practical activities. While the programme has developed from working with children with persisting speech difficulties arising from a structural abnormality (cleft lip and palate), it transcends medical diagnoses. Its principles can be used for most children from around the age of 8 years, regardless of the origin of their speech difficulties. Mixing children with a range of speech difficulties on the same course challenges the notion of condition-specific intervention and is an exciting prospect. The approach and materials could also be used in a non-residential context, but should ideally be used on an intensive basis. This programme is a major contribution to our resources for managing the unfolding nature of speech and language difficulties and should be essential reading for students and practitioners. It tackles a fundamental issue in therapy: how to bring about positive change in children with persisting communication difficulties. I look forward to using it.

Joy Stackhouse, PhD
University of Sheffield, UK.

Acknowledgements

We would like to take this opportunity to thank those who have enabled this publication to go ahead. We wish to remember the children and their parents/carers who have already participated in our intervention programme, and taught us so much. We owe a great debt of gratitude to Mrs Beryl Kellow, former Director of Speech and Language Therapy Services, Wiltshire and Swindon Health Care NHS Trust, whose enthusiasm and continuous support helped to inspire the initial study.

We wish to acknowledge the particular support and interest offered to the research team by Professor Margaret Snowling (University of York) and Professor Joy Stackhouse (University of Sheffield).

We are very grateful to The Equitable Charitable Trust who have continued to fund the research study.

PN would like to thank Robin and the boys especially, for their patience and understanding, without which this publication could not have been completed.

Introduction and background

In the social world in which we live we need the capacity to read social situations and respond appropriately to the myriad signals that human beings emit. This can mean the difference between popularity and loneliness and can smooth the route to professional and social success. We need others to satisfy both our emotional and biological needs and therefore person-to-person communication is one of the most essential human abilities. (Rustin and Kuhr, 1999, p. 3)

Introduction

This book is concerned with the management of persistent communication difficulties in school-aged children, and is presented in two parts. Part I discusses the theoretical framework which underpins the management approach being promoted and also provides an introduction to the resource material in Part II. After the introduction and background (Chapter 1), we consider how an alternative working philosophy can be put into practice (Chapter 2). Chapter 3 gives the background to the development of the resource material, and the implementation of material and a range of related activities are described in detail in Chapter 4. Part I closes with a section giving details of further reading and resources.

The resource material in Part II was developed by the research team in conjunction with residential intervention programmes devised for children with persistent communication difficulties (as discussed later in this chapter). The material is organised into several sections, and the suggested activities can either be used in the proposed chronological sequence, or can be selected as appropriate to a child's needs.

In this chapter, the primary focus is on identifying what constitutes a persistent communication difficulty, and what this means for the people concerned. An alternative means of managing dysfunctional communication in school-aged children is then examined. Particular reference is made to communication difficulties associated with cleft palate, since this is the client group with whom we initially worked. This is also a discrete group, known to experience long-term communication problems. Indeed, some young people require intermittent cleft-related treatment spanning a period of 20 years or more (e.g. Nash, 1995). The chapter ends with a discussion of why the management approach can be expanded to include other groups of communicatively-impaired children.

In the quotation above, Rustin and Kuhr (1999, p. 3) refer to 'person-to-person communication' as 'one of the most essential human abilities', and they allude to all the advantages the capacity to communicate brings in its wake. This book is concerned with the disadvantages associated with the inability to communicate effectively with others, where the 'myriad signals' are not read or responded to appropriately. Where person-to-person communication is dysfunctional, an individual's emotional and biological needs may not be met. This can lead to loneliness, and the route to social or professional success is likely to be, at the very least, a bumpy one.

It is notable that although Rustin and Kuhr refer to communication as an 'essential' ability, there is no reference to 'speech'. One explanation for this is that the term 'communication' incorporates speech. However, a more subtle interpretation may be that we are able to communicate without speech. Although speech is the most effective and rapid means of communication, communication does not necessarily depend on speech. Nevertheless, the vast majority of people are able to enjoy communicating verbally by means of speech, and ideally this capacity should be 'available' to all.

This book is based on the work of a team of experienced and specialist speech and language therapists, who are united in their pursuit for a total management approach to long-term communication difficulties. We are especially concerned with the assumptions that underlie speech and language therapy. We are also interested in asking afresh some burning questions about the priorities of intervention. What are we really expecting or hoping to achieve in our therapy? Although the current demand on clinicians within the medical model is to attend to the relevant 'diagnostic' category in managing pressurised caseloads, do we need to change the focus away from diagnosis and on to the child's daily experience of living with the difficulty, in order to effect sustained improvement?

Furthermore, do we need to stop emphasising the concept of 'good speech' as if we were expecting our patients or clients to attain 'perfect' speech, with all the ambiguity and anxiety that this perception may bring for a child? In this context, we will suggest why communication is more than speech, and how this relates to the objectives of speech and language therapy. One needs only to tap into psychological literature to appreciate the significance of communication skills. Integral to communication are the 'essential ingredients' of living in a community, relating to each other, building friendships, enjoying emotional and psychological well-being and adaptive coping skills. Indeed, there are countless references to the significance of communication breakdown in its various forms.

What is a persistent communication difficulty?

For the purposes of this book, a persistent communication difficulty comprises three distinct characteristics:

- The difficulty has continued past the age of school entry (usually 4–5 years of age).
- Progress in resolving the difficulty has

plateaued (spontaneous or 'managed' progress).
- The child has become demotivated and at risk for associated psychosocial difficulties.

Once a child has started school, it is more realistic to consider the 'original' speech and language problem as a wider communication problem. Given the nature of school life and the significant role played by peers, this can lead in turn to psychosocial difficulties (such as low self-esteem). Before pursuing this discussion, we need to consider further the implications of long-term communication impairment, both for the child and for those responsible for managing the problem.

The classification schema promoted by the World Health Organization (WHO, 1980) states: 'Impairments relate to any loss or abnormality of . . . function. Disabilities may be defined as the 'consequence of an impairment'. Handicaps more generally refer to the 'social disadvantage of a disability' and may limit or prevent the fulfillment of normal roles (Liptak, 1987).' (Eiser, 1993, p. 14). The use and relevance of these terms may be controversial in the context of a persistent communication difficulty. However, in considering the daily experience of the difficulty, it is possible, even likely, that the child has to contend with the consequences of impairment (disabilities) and the social disadvantage associated with these consequences (handicaps). Such evidence will become increasingly apparent in the subsequent pages.

Does persistent mean chronic?

Although labels can be limiting, the more precise description of some difficulties can help to identify appropriate management priorities, and to encourage more realistic expectations regarding the resolution of those difficulties. Given the long-standing nature of some communication difficulties, it may, therefore, be in a child's interests to view a persistent communication difficulty as a chronic condition, since the term chronic means 'persisting for a long time'. If such a term is accepted, the implications could be seen as advantageous to those concerned, because it:

- tempers the speech and language therapist's expectations and objectives for therapy
- necessitates a different perspective on therapy, leading to a 'total' management approach
- exposes a need to help the child adopt a realistic perspective regarding therapy
- requires a consideration of the literature on coping strategies for living with a chronic condition.

We may also accept an alternative description of a persisting communication difficulty as 'chronic communication dysfunction'. In this way, those responsible for managing the impairment are encouraged to take a wider perspective, and to see the difficulty as something that affects every aspect of the child's daily experience, rather than a discrete difficulty with a particular feature of speech.

Once we accept the terms 'chronic', and 'dysfunctional', we can legitimately make use of the growing literature on chronic conditions, which focuses on the everyday implications of living with a difficulty. It also directly addresses the wider issues and implications as they affect different family members, such that the focus is not only on the individual experiencing the difficulty, but on all those with whom that child interacts on a daily basis. A further advantage is the practical advice the literature offers on how to cope with a chronic condition. This has direct relevance for coping strategies – handling bullying at school, for example. A caveat is required here; care is needed in inadvertently alluding to associations with chronic disease or illness (such as diabetes, asthma and epilepsy), since the communicatively-impaired child is not ill or sick. Therefore, reference needs to be made only to sharing experiences of having a chronic 'condition' rather than a chronic disease.

Having looked at the rationale for describing a persistent communication difficulty as a chronic condition, we can now further develop the definition given earlier. It is now proposed that the characteristics can also be seen as defining a communication difficulty that is at risk of becoming a chronic condition, unless appropriate intervention is provided for the child concerned.

In examining the implications of living with a chronic condition, Eiser (1993) refers to the relevance of social ecology theory, which emphasises the significance of the social context in influencing how children respond to their situation. Social context includes the individual's close and extended family, and wider societal groups such as the neighbourhood, school, and hospital or clinic (where treatment is received). This can be denoted as a series of concentric rings representing the various environments with which the child interacts. The child is situated at the centre of the nested circles (Bronfenbrenner, 1979).

'The innermost ring represents the family, or 'microsystem'. This is followed by the 'mesosystem' or smaller settings, such as school or hospital where the child interacts. Third, the 'exosystem', includes settings which do not include the child directly but influence the child through family members. Included in this category would be parents' work-colleagues or friends, as well as friends and teachers of siblings.' (Eiser, 1993, p. 27).

The final level, the 'macrosystem', refers to the values and ideologies of the culture in which the child lives, which determine what happens at the other levels of Bronfenbrenner's model. In considering the relevance of the model for management of impaired communication, Dockrell and Messer (1999, p. 140) suggest: 'To be effective, interventions need to take into account the different contexts in which the child is functioning and the ways in which the difficulties the child is experiencing impact on that context.'

How the research evolved

With respect to the need to take the diversity of a child's social context into account, Stengelhofen (1993) highlights the close relationship that exists between speech and communication. As will become apparent, this relationship is a key factor in determining how effectively and competently the child is able to interact with others in different contexts.

'Any intervention to improve speech and thus enhance the individual's self-image should lead to better communication, while management to improve self-image and the development of communication skills may in fact lead to an improvement of functional speech. The interactions between these areas therefore need to be carefully evaluated, especially by the speech clinician. Team management can then be targeted on those aspects which are considered to be central in causing or maintaining the communication problems at all levels' (Stengelhofen, 1993, p. 28). As Stengelhofen suggests, improvement in speech may require attention to other factors, such as the child's self-image. It is attention to these 'other' factors that constitutes a 'total' approach to communication.

Our initial concern was to examine the persisting communication problems of older children born with cleft palate. (Hereafter the term 'cleft palate' incorporates those with cleft lip and palate and non-cleft velopharyngeal incompetence [VPI].). Cleft palate is a congenital malformation which may or may not be accompanied by additional cleft lip (unilateral or bilateral cleft lip and palate). In the UK, approximately 15 000 cleft-impaired patients need help at any one time (Enderby and Philipp, 1986). In speech terms, cleft palate is recognised as a 'structural disorder' of the vocal tract (Albery, 1986, p. 52). Cleft palate can profoundly affect speech development, but cleft lip does not usually cause speech difficulties.

The majority of children with cleft lip and palate develop satisfactory communication after surgery. However, around 40% of cases have persisting difficulties that lead to deficits in communication skills (Stengelhofen, 1993). VPI can also cause major speech problems in the absence of a cleft, since efficient functioning of the velopharynx is integral to normal speech production. VPI-related speech difficulties share many of the features of 'cleft speech', the majority of which can be improved with a combination of surgery and speech and language therapy (Stengelhofen, 1993, p. 5). For a fuller account of the management and psychosocial implications of persistent communication difficulties associated with cleft palate, the reader is referred to Nash (1995) and Nash et al. (2001b).

Even after expert surgery, some children with cleft palate or VPI will still require speech and language therapy after entering school, with long-term implications for their psychosocial welfare (e.g. Stengelhofen, 1993; Nash, 1995). Although some of these children will achieve good communication, others will require help during adolescence and beyond. The progress of children in this latter group may plateau for various reasons: for example, special education needs, hearing loss, malocclusion, or a long wait for further surgical or orthodontic treatment. A minority of young people do not receive the necessary treatment because they (or their parents) do not attend speech and language therapy appointments.

A further explanation for persisting communication problems may be that children are not receiving the necessary psychosocial help within their clinical management, since speech and language impairment frequently implicates a wider communication difficulty. Whatever the reason, those concerned must be helped to cope with their long-term difficulties, by incorporating attention to psychosocial aspects within their clinical management. Some clinicians and school teachers may, however, believe that it is not their responsibility to provide psychosocial help within the confines of a busy caseload or classroom. Ideally, help should be offered at a time that avoids disruption of schooling. This will be discussed further in Chapters 2 and 3.

A closer look at the implications of school-aged children receiving speech and language therapy shows that the longer they require help, the more schooling they miss and the more likely they are to be victimised and stigmatised by peers for being 'different'. This is especially evident where a child has to leave the school classroom for a clinical appointment, and is labelled by peers for doing so. It also reinforces the child's self-perception as someone who has a 'problem' significant enough to miss lessons. A vicious circle can ensue which contributes to the child's cycle of disadvantage (Nash, 1995; Nash et al., 2001b).

Our research study focused on the plight of children with a history of cleft palate aged 8–18 years, who for one reason or another had plateaued in their progress in communication ('children' hereafter denotes both children and adolescents). That is, although they have received excellent surgery and the equivalent of many hours of individual speech and language therapy over many years, they appear not to reflect the result of so much professional attention. In these cost-conscious days we need to ask why there is relatively so little to show for so much investment of time and energy. Indeed, in view of the sometimes lengthy treatment programme, Kapp-Simon et al. (1992) include young people with cleft palate in their study of children with chronic physical conditions.

Psychosocial implications of persistent communication difficulties

For children with persistent communication difficulties, sounding and possibly looking different from peers (for example, having a cleft lip and palate) has a potential psychological impact that cannot be underestimated. Indeed, such children are at risk for victimisation, and often display the 'teasing complex' (Gerrard, 1991), whereby those who are teased become progressively more withdrawn and distressed. They may also exhibit 'communication apprehension' (McCroskey and Beatty, 1984), indicating fear or anxiety associated with communicating with others. Attention to psychosocial factors alongside work on communication can, therefore, greatly enhance communication competence and social integration. Unless some form of intervention is offered, dysfunctional patterns of behaviour often persist into adulthood (e.g. Stengelhofen, 1993; Nash, 1995).

In the case of cleft lip and palate, self-consciousness about facial disfigurement can also cause psychosocial difficulties such as poor interpersonal communication skills and low self-esteem (for instance, Kapp-Simon and McGuire, 1997). Therefore, from birth, children with cleft lip and palate are considered to be especially 'at risk' of developing dysfunctional communication.

Chesebro et al. (1992, p. 353) have noted the potentially adverse effects of schooling for the cleft-impaired, which have wider implications for all those with persistent communication difficulties:

'Since much of the communication between students and teachers in the classroom must be student-initiated . . . it is probable that students who feel communicatively inadequate do not engage in many of the important learning activities available in the class.'

Summary of research to date

In considering how to address the obvious need for some form of psychosocial intervention, we devised a programme that focuses on the total communication needs of the participants, by means of intensive residential group work. Favourable outcomes of projects based on offering intensive speech therapy to groups of children with cleft palate have already been reported by Albery and Chapman (1979) and Huskie (1979), among others. These interventions were primarily aimed at improving the children's speech.

The current intervention programme incorporates psychosocial, cognitive and emotional dimensions of communication, with attention to speech features and oral communication. It encompasses strategies for coping with bullying and enhancing self-esteem, and assertiveness training. The programme also focuses on listening skills, phonetic and phonological levels of speech, the use of 'best' speech and social skills. Individual and group activities are included on all aspects of the children's identified needs. Although the emphasis is on group work in a natural environment, the generalisation of individually achieved objectives is encouraged within the various group activities.

To date, we have run two residential intervention programmes and undertaken a national survey on the extent of persistent communication difficulties associated with cleft palate in children 8–18 years of age. The first intervention programme (1996) was carried out as a pilot study. As a result of concern over the serious nature of the participants' persisting communication difficulties, we conducted a national postal survey to look at the size of the problem on a national scale. The survey was followed by a second residential intervention programme in 1999. Details as to how the research study is being currently expanded are given later in the chapter.

Piloting the residential intervention programme

The residential intervention programme was piloted in August 1996, and was offered over a period of 1 week to eight children with cleft palate (or VPI) whose progress in communication had plateaued. The venue for the week was a tailor-made annexe attached to a residential school in Wiltshire, which is used for a wide variety of children's programmes. Accommodation and activity sessions took place under one roof, which made arrangements considerably more convenient. The annexe was surrounded by a large open space, fenced off from the road, which the children enjoyed during free times. It proved to be an ideal and conducive environment in which to run the programme.

The children taking part were aged 9–15 years (mean age 12.6 years; four male, four female). At post-intervention assessment 10 weeks later, there was evidence of notable improvements in communication in all of the participants. The most marked progress for all children was enhanced self-confidence in speaking out and increased ability to listen to others. The youngsters also held more positive perceptions of themselves and their capabilities, including voicing their anxieties about communication. The pilot study is reported in full by Nash et al. (1997).

The national survey

The pilot study raised concerns about the national scale of persisting communication problems. These concerns became the prime reason for developing the study, with the support of further research funding from The Equitable Charitable Trust. The first objective of the study was to examine the prevalence of persistent communication difficulties associated with cleft palate in school-aged children.

Nash et al. (2001c) undertook a national postal survey which was sent to all 206 NHS speech and language therapy managers or directors in England and Wales, to identify young people aged 8–18 with cleft palate who had persisting communication difficulties. The high response rate to the survey (148 replies; 71.8%), may indicate an area of largely unmet need. The findings show that a number of children still experience persistent communication problems in middle childhood and beyond. That is, from a total of 80 (38.8%) NHS Trusts returning completed forms, 303 children were identified as having long-term communication problems. Twelve of these individuals were studied further by attending a residential intervention programme (July 1999, outlined below). Blank forms were received from 55 (26.7%) respondents, indicating that they did not know of any such children. A further 13 (6.3%) respondents made contact by telephone or mail to say either that the information was coming in due course, or that they were unable to access the required details by the specified deadline. There were 58 (28.2%) non-respondents overall. The findings of the survey have far-reaching implications for all involved in the management of the children's psychosocial welfare (especially the hospital-based Cleft Palate Team), and those responsible for their education.

Implications of national survey findings

An examination of the survey data indicates that there is considerable variation in the respondents' level and depth of knowledge of the children concerned. For example, although the large majority of respondents provided full details on questions concerning speech and language, we need to ask why over one-third of them (102 respondents, 33.7%) reported that they did not know whether or not a child was or had been subjected to teasing and bullying by others. Do we not know because we do not specifically ask children about their daily experiences of living with persistent communication difficulties? Do we not ask them because we feel that there is no help available even if the answer is yes, or because we think it is not relevant to facilitating progress? There is little doubt about the pressure speech and language therapists are under to manage ever-increasing caseloads. When treating a child's communication problem, however, the way in which the youngster functions in everyday life must be of crucial interest to the clinician in managing that difficulty.

In sum, the high response rate to the postal survey not only reflects the respondents' support, but appears to unveil an area of largely unmet need. On this occasion, the study focused specifically on youngsters with cleft palate or VPI. One can only guess at the enormous scale of the problem if the psychosocial needs of all communicatively-impaired children and adolescents were taken into consideration. We plan to conduct a further national survey to include all school-aged children with persisting communication difficulties. It is hoped that a clearer picture will then emerge of the true size of the problem and the potential impact of such difficulties for the children concerned.

The residential intervention programme

Following the success of the pilot study, 206 NHS speech and language therapy directors or managers were invited to identify by means of a national survey (outlined below), any children whom they thought might benefit from attending a residential intervention programme. A total of 67 (22.1%) referral forms were subsequently sent out to collect information on the children concerned, and 19 forms were completed and returned. These referral forms were then examined in conjunction with the selection criteria for inclusion in the July 1999 programme (Table 1.1), which focused on the impact of the cleft (or VPI) on the child's communication abilities and level of need. The tight deadline that

had to be imposed for the return of the forms may account for the relatively small return rate.

Assessment

Fourteen children fulfilled the selection criteria (Nash et al., 2001c), and were invited for assessment in May 1999. All aspects of the programme (assessment, intervention, and follow-up) were scheduled to take place in the school holidays. Pre-intervention assessment of the potential participants was undertaken 9 weeks before the intervention programme (May), and post-intervention assessment took place 10 weeks after the programme (October). The children were also assessed immediately after completion of the intervention (July). The same assessments were administered on each occasion. At the post-intervention assessment, the children and their parents or caregivers were asked to complete an evaluation form.

In conjunction with the objectives for the residential programme, assessment focused on psychosocial functioning and speech and language, and comprised the following measures:

Psychosocial functioning
The Emotional Behaviour Scales (EBS, Clarbour and Roger, 1999) developed at the University of York incorporate three scales that tap

Table 1.1 Criteria for selection of participants to attend residential programme

Age within specified band (8–18 years old)

Cleft palate (with/out additional cleft lip) or VPI

Child has been/continues to be subjected to teasing/bullying

Child's persistent communication difficulties have psychosocial implications (i.e. social skills and relationships with friends adversely affected)

Child's low self-esteem and self-confidence is adversely affecting competence as an effective communicator

Intelligibility rating of 1–4 (according to CAPS, Harding et al., 1996)

Child is self-conscious about speech or appearance

Child does not have severe language delay or severe learning difficulties (due to demands of residential programme and feeling of well-being within group)

Child can be fully assessed before and after intervention

Referring speech and language therapist thinks child might benefit from attendance because of the intensive nature of the residential programme

Child is prepared to attend programme without parents/caregiver

into anxiety about relating to others, self-esteem and experiences of being bullied by other children:

1   Social Anxiety
2   Social Self-Esteem
3   Malevolent Aggression

Speech and language
(complete video and audio recordings were made)

- Sentences common to Great Ormond Street Speech Assessment (GOS.SP.ASS. '98, Sell et al., 1999) and Cleft Audit Protocol for Speech (CAPS – Harding et al., 1996).
- Spontaneous speech sample in which child views and retells story of a well-known video.
- One-to-one discussion with child around six questions to explore feelings about speech, being understood by others, having to work on speech change, insights into the speech process and level of awareness of their communication.
- An oral examination was carried out as appropriate.

Although CAPS (above) lists the resonatory, nasal emission and voice aspects, these were not listed as separate needs on this occasion, because the team felt that these parameters cannot be successfully handled separately from other areas, such as speaking out, articulation and the suprasegmental aspects of speech. Indeed, aspects such as rate, volume and intonation were considered of prime importance in bringing about change, and they were interwoven with all the work undertaken with the children. That is, we believe that the achievement of balanced resonance and reducing nasal emission, as well as the reduction of dysphonia, is a by-product of using the larynx and vocal tract in a balanced and non-abusive way.

This point is of importance because when the referring therapists were asked on the referral form: 'What aspects of the child's speech do you see as problematic?', none of them mentioned dysphonia, which the team identified in six

children, being very severe in three cases. This is closely related to hypernasality and abusive articulatory patterns, such as glottalisation. In devising priorities for speech and language therapy, it is possible that we may continue to work on features of speech that are persisting failures for the child, and which may actually be undermining the individual's self-confidence.

During the assessment, while one speech and language therapist was interviewing the child, another watched with the parents through a one-way viewing screen. This method provided the opportunity to collect more information on the child's history, progress, and day-to-day communication and for parents to express their concerns. To supplement the more formal data collection, the children were also observed while playing and interacting with the other children and their parents; notes were made on their social interaction.

After the initial assessment, 12 children were invited to attend the residential programme, all of whom accepted. The group had the following profile:

- 3 females and 9 males
- aged 8–14 years (mean age 11.2 years)
- from a wide geographical spread
- presented with cleft lip and palate (unilateral or bilateral, n = 7), cleft of the soft palate only (n = 3) or VPI (n = 2).
- When referred, 7 children were receiving regular speech and language therapy, and 5 were on review.

Once we had established which children would be participating in the programme, a postal questionnaire was sent to their respective headteachers to gather information about the participants' school life. A total of 9 (75%) forms were subsequently completed and returned, providing valuable insights into how the individuals coped at school on a daily basis.

In conjunction with the research design, the referring speech and language therapists agreed to suspend all speech and language therapy intervention in the period between pre- and post-intervention assessment of the children (i.e. May–October 1999).

At the start of the intervention programme, objectives derived from assessment were discussed with each child and their parents or caregiver, and reviewed again with them at the end of the course. In planning the activities for the week, due consideration was given to the need to establish a 'safe' and supportive environment for the children so that they felt enabled to address sensitive issues. As the same venue was used as in the pilot intervention, we were confident that such an environment would be provided.

Apart from the use of electropalatography (EPG), the methods used did not depend on high technological expertise, and were within the skills of all speech and language therapists. We believe that nearly all aspects of communication change can be carried out in a group setting, ideally with therapists and children working together and creating a natural, non-pressurised situation. This has implications for cost-effectiveness, as well as professional development.

Findings after the residential intervention programme

After the post-intervention assessment, a full report was sent to each child's referring speech and language therapist, which provided feedback and recommendations for ways forward, based on the child's progress during the week.

Feedback from participants and their parents at post-intervention, 10 weeks later, showed evidence of notable improvements in communication in all participants. The most sustained improvement for all children was greater self-confidence in speaking out and listening skills. Children also reported a positive change in relations with peers, and had established good friendships at school. The participants were clearly more enabled to perceive themselves in a new light and to voice their anxieties about communication. It was also evident that all the children had begun to change the perception of themselves as communicators – a key to further progress. It is noteworthy that there were close similarities in the nature of the improvements sustained by the children

attending the two intervention programmes (1996 and 1999).

Findings relating to the psychosocial assessment of the participants, as measured by the Emotional Behaviour Scales (Clarbour and Roger, 1999), suggest positive changes in the dimensions of social anxiety, social self-esteem and malevolent aggression. Further findings of this intervention study are reported by Nash et al. (2001b).

Evaluation received from participating children and parents or caregivers

The following comments have been selected from among those received after the two intervention programmes (1996 and 1999). It is interesting to note that the four 'themes' arising from the follow-up data, were precisely the areas identified as key objectives for the residential programme. The four 'themes' were:

* increased self-confidence
* improved speech
* more rewarding friendships
* use of effective coping strategies.

Spontaneous feedback at 8 weeks post intervention

One child spontaneously wrote a letter 8 weeks post-intervention about the week away. This participant had found it '. . . better talking to the group than school because we all had the same problem so we found it easier talking in a group'. After a long history of being teased by classmates, this child noted that the week '. . . (has) made me a different person, you made me face the others who are normal. When people call me names it does not hurt me much and that was the most important thing for me because I really wanted to get on with my work and my life.'

Follow-up at 10 weeks post-intervention assessment
Selection of feedback from participating children

* I enjoyed the work we did in the daytime and I think it made everyone happier because we could share our feelings.
* My brother said that my speech is getting

better each time (I practise), and if I keep doing it I will get even better.

- It made me think I've got a few friends.
- I've made friends quicker.

Selection of feedback from parents or caregivers

- Before holiday he was saying he had no friends, now he doesn't say this. He needed someone to listen to him.
- He was bullied every day, locked in toilets etc., not happening now.
- Now mixing in a group of children, before (intervention) was only confident with adults.
- It brought her out of herself . . . communication has come on a lot.

Follow-up at 12 months post-intervention

The purpose of the follow-up postal questionnaire was to monitor the children's progress 1 year after attending the 1999 residential programme. This was in addition to the follow-up questionnaires at 3 and 6 months post-intervention. Eight of the 12 (66.7%) questionnaires sent out were completed and returned. The responses reflected a positive profile regarding the maintenance of progress and continued motivation to practise the recommendations we made during the residential programme. Further follow-up data is reported in Nash et al. (2001c).

Selection of feedback from participating children

a)   Can you remember what was the most helpful/ most important thing for you during the week?

- Learning how to cope with bullies and teasing.
- Yes, I read out loud in class and feel happier about my speech.
- I learnt loads of new sounds. I talk slower and don't get so muddled.
- People are beginning to understand me better when I talk, people don't pick on me so much.
- I feel confident now and better about my speech and the way I look, it was good meeting other children like me.

b)   Looking back, did the holiday week make any difference to the way you NOW feel?

- More sure of (my)self.
- Doesn't take so long to make friends.
- Now other people can understand my speech.
- In school lesson I speak with a loud and clear voice.
- Yes. Not so nervous when going somewhere for the first time.

Selection of feedback from parents or caregivers

a)   Looking back, have any changes which you noticed in your child's speech after the course last summer been maintained?

- Still speaking out and standing up to bullies.
- Yes in all ways and he continues to improve.
- Yes . . . He speaks more clearly.
- Yes, at X's statement review, his teacher stated how much confidence he has now, and how well he got on with the rest of his class, and how well he contributed to questions asked about the things they were doing at school, and how pleased the other children were with X's contribution.

b)   Looking back, do you think the holiday week made any difference to the way X NOW feels?

- More people understand X now and his confidence is oozing.
- Yes, he is more confident in all ways.
- Other people have said he was easier to understand after (the week away).
- Yes. X lost his sense of isolation. X was also able to benefit from spending time with people who understood his condition.
- X is more confident and able to approach others to form mutually beneficial relationships.
- Yes. X's knowledge that 'he is not alone' has certainly helped. He has grown in confidence.
- He is more confident now and contributes to the work at school and the

rest of his class have been pleased with his contribution.

A speech and language therapist who had referred a child for the residential programme offered her first impressions on meeting the child again after attending the programme:

'The first thing that struck me was the confidence X exuded, having been previously rather withdrawn (and at times, monosyllabic) ... Teasing does not bother X now ... I feel a huge amount has been achieved for X in a relatively short space of time. Addressing all the concerns that X had could not have been achieved in the clinic situation. X's speech is now much more readily intelligible, but above all she feels good about herself and I cannot ever remember X feeling that way before.'

Discussion of findings after the intervention programme

The experience of living with the children for a week raised many questions about the discrepancy that often exists between the child's 'best' and everyday speech. Indeed, the speech a child produces during a relatively short speech assessment may not be an accurate reflection of his or her functional speech. As a result, objectives and expectations regarding subsequent speech improvements may be built on a false picture of the child's abilities. A far clearer picture may be obtained by adopting more flexibility in speech assessments. The value of this became increasingly evident during the pre- and post-intervention assessments, when we all agreed that the children's speech should have been monitored throughout the day, not just for a small proportion of it. The large sample of free speech collected during pre- and post-intervention assessment, by the re-telling of a well-known video story, went some way towards obtaining a representative sample.

The study suggests that learning to be a competent and effective communicator is more pertinent to a child's psychosocial welfare and quality of life than continuing to pursue improved speech, which may not only be unattainable but may also adversely affect a child's perception of his or her own capabilities. We therefore have a responsibility to find ways of moving these young people forward. The study supports the view that an intensive residential holiday situation, shared with other children with similar problems, provides opportunity for multidimensional intervention of a unique nature which can be the key to change. Further details of the residential intervention programme are given in Chapter 3.

Post-intervention liaison with referring speech and language therapists

After the post-intervention assessment, we held a 1-day meeting with the speech and language therapists of children who had attended the programme. Nine therapists (75%) attended the day. The objective of the day was to discuss the implications of the programme with the therapists, with specific reference to the children they had referred. The meeting also offered the opportunity to explore principles of intervention and general management of persistent communication difficulties.

At the end of the meeting, the participating speech and language therapists were asked to address what had been learned about:

1. an individual child's progress
2. principles of intervention
   (any you felt you might like to pursue)
3. management alternatives

Sample of comments from referring speech and language therapists attending meeting to discuss the July 1999 programme:

1. What have we learned about an individual child's progress?
- An individual's progress focused on other factors, e.g. dysphonia (voice aspects) and bullying.
- Progress is as much dependent on 'speaking out' and self-esteem, as on actual articulation work.
- Progress must be measured on many fronts, not 'simply' speech production – the overspill from one lift in self-esteem can be enormous.

- What a week can achieve, e.g. confidence and clarity. Reducing tension and speaking out can improve the whole communication of the child.

2. Principles of intervention
(any you felt you might like to pursue)

- Intervention is a 'multi-faceted' problem; must be multidimensional too.
- Look more at breathing, relaxation techniques.
- Work more in groups and informal setting.
- Need to look more at e.g. relaxation/ posture not just articulation, and psychosocial issues, holistic approach.
- Articulation work hand in hand with confidence building in a supportive 'team' setting, with real opportunities for reinforcement and generalisation.

3. Management alternatives

- I think I should consider how to put children together, rather than working in isolation.
- Relating other client groups together, e.g. relaxation in groups.
- Running 'speaking out' group for children with different problems.
- The use of a broad range of activities, not focusing on one area.

The participants identified many key issues, and were clearly enthusiastic about the approach being proposed for the management of persisting communication difficulties. We are looking forward to further collaboration with other speech and language therapists, with the future extension of the research project.

Why the research study can be expanded to include other groups

Although the initial study focused on children with communication difficulties associated with a history of cleft palate, it has become increasingly apparent to us that many of the difficulties experienced are precisely those that characterise persistent communication impairment. That is, alongside the specific cleft-related speech difficulties, the children displayed a variety of problems of a psychosocial nature (such as low self-esteem, poor self-image, few friends). It is proposed that such problems, in turn, are a feature of having to cope with dysfunctional communication at school, where a child is no longer buffered by the nurturing environment of the pre-school years. It is also at school that the pivotal role of peers becomes ever more significant, which in itself heralds a set of potential new challenges for those with communication difficulties (such as bullying). It is for these reasons that our working philosophy (outlined above) has direct application and scope for encompassing into the research study other groups of children with persistent communication difficulties.

There is a notable shortage of literature on the psychosocial implications of living with a speech impairment (articulatory, phonetic or phonological), although there is 'ample evidence of adverse social consequences' related to language impairment (Bishop, 1997, p. 213). We do know that some children in mainstream education have phonological impairment, and that this may be in association with other spoken and written language 'deficits' including dyslexia. The association between poor literacy skills and speech difficulties is now well documented (for example, Stackhouse and Wells, 1998; Snowling et al., 1999). Such impairment can seriously hamper a child's expressive communication. Therefore, it seems probable that this difficulty is noticed by peers, and if seen as something sufficiently different by them, may invite ridicule and other forms of bullying.

In his cross-national investigation of school bullying, Smith (1999, p. 73) notes that several studies indicate that children with special educational needs are: 'substantially more at risk of being involved in bully/victim situations'. This group of children included a wide range of physical, emotional, behavioural and learning disabilities, including dyslexia.

Although there is sparse literature on the incidence of bullying amongst speech and language-impaired children, the area is attracting growing interest. For instance, Mooney and Smith (1995, p.26) refer to bullying as: 'a very real problem' for dysfluent children. They point out that although speech and language therapy may reduce dysfluency, the prognosis is less optimistic after about seven years of age and the difficulty may persist into adulthood. As with all forms of expressive communication impairment, a child's schooling may also be coloured by adverse experiences related to dysfluency.

The short and long-term impact of bullying can be very profound, such as loss of self-confidence and self-esteem, increased anxiety and shyness and problems with making friends. 'Children who stammer are often shy and anxious in social settings, and this may be heightened by anxiety over possibly imminent bullying. ... If a child is worrying about bullying in the school ... or after school, it is likely that his or her self-esteem and academic work will suffer. ... It seems that it is not only their self-confidence that can be affected, but also their home-life, friends and school work' (Mooney and Smith, 1995, p. 24-25). It is also probable that dysfluent children are not able to assert themselves when subjected to bullying, if they do not possess the necessary coping or social skills to deflect the situation.

Mooney and Smith (1995) note that the bullying of dysfluent children is reported by many speech and language therapists, especially in the form of ridicule and name-calling. The high incidence of bullying is endorsed by their finding that in a postal questionnaire, 82% of respondents (n=324) reported that they had been subjected to bullying at some stage at school. Bullying was most prevalent between 11-13 years old (39%), and then in 8-10 year olds (27%).

In highlighting the repercussions of being bullied for the dysfluent child, the authors go on to assert that such experiences may become the most significant feature of his/her life. Bullying appears to have long-term consequences for some children, who, as adults may become nervous and anxious, fearing ridicule by other people and finding socialising difficult. According to Mooney and Smith, some dysfluent adults believe that bullying has tended to make them more aggressive.

Frequent victimisation of children with persistent communication difficulties has been cited by Nash (1995), who found that 80.2% of the 174 cleft-impaired children studied reported being teased or bullied. Young people with persistent communication difficulties may be especially susceptible to bullying, partly because they are perceived by their peers as not having the appropriate social skills to handle bullying effectively.

In the context of language impairment, Bishop (1997, p. 214) notes that children with limited language skills are at a high risk for being rejected by peers. For example, Rice et al. (1991) showed that pre-school children are sensitive to their peers' communicative status, such that they tend not to initiate social inter-action with those who have limited language skills. Rice et al. also report that pre-school children speaking a foreign language similarly experienced difficulties with being accepted by peers. This finding endorses the theory that children's reactions to their peers are deter-mined by how a child communicates, rather than any underlying social limitations (Bishop, 1997).

There also appears to be little research on the self-perceptions of communicatively-impaired children. Lindsay and Dockrell (2000, p. 585) note:

'These children may be considered likely to have more negative self perceptions for three reasons; firstly, the effects of failure at school and associated negative feedback; secondly the stigmatising effects of being singled out and labelled; and thirdly effects specific to the nature of communication difficulties.'

They refer to the reciprocal relationship between self-perception and performance, which effects a self-fulfilling prophecy. That is, the 'successful' child, in terms of school performance and personal relationships, is likely to be motivated and successful which, in turn, fuel a positive self-perception (for example, Blatchford, 1992). Conversely, children who harbour a negative self-perception of their own capabilities and social competence, may be less 'successful' in these areas, which can result in demotivation and lower levels of achievement.

Stengelhofen (1993, p. 28) cites examples of dysfunctional communication from her personal clinical experience. Adolescents with a cleft were 'extremely reluctant to communicate in most situations', and displayed characteristic behaviours such as avoiding situations where they would be required to talk, avoiding eye contact by hiding behind their hair, lowering their head and using low intensity and fast paced speech. Contrary to their intentions, these individuals draw attention to themselves by their whole demeanour and unintelligible speech, which may be worsened by features that distract the listener (for example, nasal grimace). Thus, anxiety about speech adversely affects appearance, and anxieties about appearance disturb the flow of communication.

Thomas et al. (1997, p. 226) stress that an individual's self-esteem and satisfaction with personal appearance may be more significant in determining social behaviour than the degree of disfigurement. Similarly, Harter (1999, p. 158) notes that even amongst her young (4–7 year old) sample, 'physical appearance headed the list in terms of the domain most highly correlated with self-worth'. Unless some form of intervention is offered, the dysfunctional patterns of behaviour may persist into adulthood.

It is notable that alongside the vast literature on aspects of speech and language impairment, there continues to be a lack of consensus on the precise definitions and descriptions of such deficits (for example, reviews by Bishop, 1997; Hill, 2001). It is not possible to review this literature comprehensively in the limited space available, but we are aware of its relevance in any discussion of persistent communication difficulties. In identifying pertinent selection criteria for the residential programme, important questions arose concerning language impairment, since

the nature of the programme required the participants to have a certain level of language comprehension. That is, in order to benefit from the intervention, it was decided to exclude any child with severe language delay or severe learning difficulties. In reality, even where language was considered to be a secondary difficulty, the relationship between cause and effect was far from certain. Indeed, there were some indicators to suggest that the expressive language of some children was being held back by persistent speech difficulties. In light of this finding, the relationship between speech and language competence is clearly an issue that we wish to investigate in future (for example, Dockrell and Messer, 1999).

The research reported in this chapter raises some challenging management issues. What are and what should be the priorities of speech and language therapists and school teachers, when planning the management of a child with a persistent communication difficulty? Kapp-Simon and McGuire (1997, p. 380) highlight the essence of what could be seen as effective therapy: 'A socially competent individual is one who is able to generate a response to an interpersonal situation that is appropriate and meets the demands of that situation.'

In spite of the many advances in our understanding of speech and language and therapeutic techniques, the fundamental question remains: 'how do I bring about change in this child's speech?' This is a particularly burning question where the school-aged child may have already received the equivalent of many hours' therapy over the years. We suggest that the asking of this fundamental question heralds the need to switch course and to focus on the wider psychosocial aspects of the communication difficulty. It is because this question can be asked by any speech and language therapist, no matter what client group they may be managing, that the current research study can be expanded to include groups of varying aetiologies, ages and contexts (for example, non-residential intensive group work).

The next chapter introduces relevant psychological literature for insight into why we need to adopt a broader understanding of communication in managing persistent communication difficulties. It also looks at the wider psychosocial implications of the difficulties for those experiencing them, and those who are managing them.

2 Putting an alternative working philosophy into practice

'Here is Edward Bear, coming downstairs now bump, bump, on the back of his head behind Christopher Robin. It is, as far as he knows, the only way of coming downstairs, but sometimes he feels that there really is another way, if only he could stop bumping for a moment and think of it.' (A.A. Milne, Winnie the Pooh)

Adopting a broader understanding of communication

In the previous chapter we established the need to adopt a broader approach to communication. In this chapter we present the rationale and supporting evidence for incorporating psychosocial concepts into the management of persisting communication difficulties. A discussion of the working philosophy that continues to underpin our approach is followed by an examination of the role of self-esteem and self-perception in dysfunctional communication, and how these are key issues in devising effective intervention. The subsequent section introduces a conceptual framework for identifying those most at risk for psychosocial difficulties associated with dysfunctional communication. The chapter ends with consideration of coping styles, and how they help or hinder a child's ability to deal with the challenges of persistent communication difficulties on a daily basis.

The management approach being promoted is driven by a working philosophy, which encapsulates both principles and management objectives. The philosophy is presented below and subsequently 'unpicked', by way of examining the conceptual framework that underpins the holistic approach to managing persistent communication difficulties.

Our working philosophy and its implications for intervention

Speech and language deficits are disabling on two grounds; first, the communication impairment in itself, and second, because the impairment frequently leads to and/or is concurrent with psychosocial problems which involve low self-esteem and bullying or teasing, and this in turn causes further deterioration in communication. To attend to the specific speech and language deficit without also managing the wider implications is a barrier to progress and has long-term consequences for the individual in education, in social adjustment and in employment.

Our work is driven by the view that the management of the communicatively-impaired child, as a whole, must be taken into account in the 'treatment' of an identified speech and language deficit. Attention to the child's psychosocial needs, to help them to cope and to boost their self-esteem, will pave the way to enabling them to tackle their communication difficulties. As Kish and Garlick (1999, p. 8) note in their work with the facially disfigured: 'Our experience highlights the generic nature of the psycho-social needs of children with disfiguring conditions and supports a generic approach to managing these, in contrast to a medical model which offers condition-specific intervention.'

It is proposed that if a communication problem persists into the school-age years, it is confounded by another set of problems due to the very nature of the initial difficulty. For example, children whose communication impairment is still prominent when they start school (aged 4–5 years), are likely not only to have to deal with the impairment itself, but because of the social function of communication and the expectations of peers, may well also have to handle the consequences of the impairment. These consequences often mean low self-esteem, poor self-perception, and potential victimisation by peers for being perceived as 'different' from other children. These children may also be perceived (by adults as well as peers), as being 'unable', that is, as not capable of expressing themselves nor of coping effectively with particular needs.

For the school child with persisting communication difficulties, we cannot and should not, therefore, neglect the potential consequences of those difficulties. The relationship between impaired communication and psychosocial difficulties is such that the latter may actually trigger the former (as well as vice versa). Another important point to highlight is the fundamental differences between the daily experience of communication impairment during the pre-school years, compared with what happens when a child reaches school. In general, the pre-school years tend to be nurturing years spent with a primary caregiver or at playgroup or nursery, where children tend to be accepting and unquestioning over apparent differences between themselves and other children.

A very different picture emerges at school, where in accordance with the child's psychological development, differences begin to be noticed and commented on. Moreover, there is generally much less tolerance of difference, which is frequently the source of bullying at school. An individual who is deemed to be 'different' (because of size, colouring or any other characteristic), may be labelled and marginalised by peers (Erwin, 1993). Because this labelling process is inevitable, it should be possible to identify those who may be vulnerable, especially if the very means by which the child interacts and socialises is dysfunctional. Since such experiences may well exacerbate the deterioration of communication competence, there is a pressing need for the wider psychosocial implications of dysfunctional communication to be taken into consideration at the pre-school stage, and certainly when the child reaches school age. Bishop (1997, p. 209) asserts that the presence of both non-verbal and verbal communication impairment suggests that there is 'a broader underlying problem with social

communication that cannot be attributed to difficulties with oral language'.

The potential adverse consequences of having not only persistent communication difficulties, but also low self-esteem and persistent bullying by peers, must not be underestimated. The effects of these childhood experiences can stay with someone for life, and affect every aspect of their adult life. We shall return to these issues in due course.

The resource material in Part II illustrates how impaired communication can be managed as a whole, for example, by integrating work on enhancing self-esteem into a speech and language therapy framework. This approach may challenge the biomedical (or medical) model approach to therapy, since it may require an uncomfortable reappraisal of aims, objectives and priorities, which, as Kish and Garlick (1999, p. 8) suggest above, focuses on condition-specific intervention.

Biomedical vs biopsychosocial models

It is useful at this point to examine the underlying assumptions of the (bio)medical model, and to contrast them with growing interest in the (bio)psychosocial model. The comparison between these two paradigms can offer insights into the necessity of a shift of emphasis in managing school-aged children who are communicatively impaired. Sarafino (1990, p. 16) aptly describes the two predominant models of intervention:

'Once we add the person to the biomedical model, we have a different and broader picture of how health and illness come about. This new perspective involves the interplay of biological, psychological, and social aspects of the person's life ... (and) ... is called the biopsychosocial model.' (for example, Schwartz, 1982.) This model is sometimes referred to as 'holistic', a term that derives from the Greek word holos meaning 'whole' (Lipowski, 1986).

The biomedical model dominated the twentieth century, and has strong roots in cartesian dualism, which makes a clear distinction between mind and body functions. The role of biochemical factors in managing illness was considered of paramount importance, with little attention paid to the possible influence of psychosocial, social and behavioural dimensions (Engel, 1980). Sheridan and Radmacher (1992, p. 3) point out, however, that before the acceptance of cartesian dualism, great importance was attached to the part psychological factors played in determining illness and health. McClelland (1985, p. 452) has heralded the value of health psychology, and speaks of the medical model as mechanistic, in its treatment of the body as a machine that can be 'fixed' as necessary.

As discontent with the narrow framework offered by the biomedical model has grown, attention has turned to expanding the model to include a more global perspective of health. The consequent biopsychosocial model is founded on general systems theory, which assumes that nothing exists alone or in isolation. The model compels specialists to consider the 'whole' person in their management of the presenting problem. It therefore acknowledges the significance and relevance of pertinent psychological concepts, rather than underestimating or even ignoring their potential role (Sheridan and Radmacher, 1992, p. 5).

Brumfitt (1999, p. 108) endorses the priorities of the biopsychosocial model in the context of speech and language therapy: 'On meeting with a client we see a person with an individual identity but set in a family structure and influenced by other factors that arise out of growing older and experiencing good or bad health. We cannot therefore view . . . a child with a phonological impairment as nothing but a child with that problem. Each client who we meet comes with a multidimensional set of views and experiences and we need to incorporate them into our professional perception of them. We disregard them at our peril.'

A further implication of the biopsychosocial model is the distinction that can be made between providing 'treatment' and providing other forms of help or intervention in changing certain communication behaviours. The former is inherently linked with the medical model's emphasis on the process of assessment, diagnosis, treatment and prognosis, with the

conventional receptive role of the 'patient'. The latter, however, shifts the emphasis to the more proactive 'client', with whom the therapist or trainer forms a partnership role as together they explore and learn from the intervention.

The implications of the two different models for speech and language therapy can be seen in the nature of the relationship that exists (or could exist) between the clinician and the child attending the appointment. Within the medical model the clinician is seen as the expert, who has both 'the knowledge' and the expertise to affect change in the child's speech. What this message conveys to the child (and parents or caregivers) is that the clinician is in control of what the child learns, since therapy is generally prescribed according to the individual's identified needs.

The alternative to this paradigm, which derives from the biopsychosocial model, is especially conducive to managing persistent communication difficulties. In the context of this framework, children are encouraged to think about their own communication abilities and how the persistent difficulties may be affecting their life. This may take the form of engaging a child in a discussion of their perceived needs and anxieties about communicating with others, and identifying aspirations regarding communication or mixing with peers. It could also involve developing self-monitoring and self-evaluation skills as the child becomes actively involved in addressing his or her own particular areas of need. Parents and caregivers can also be drawn into discussions, where appropriate. This shift of emphasis echoes that advocated by Hopson and Scally (1981, p. 111) in the context of education, in which attention is moved from formal teaching to experiential learning '. . . with each student being given more responsibility for his own direction and development'. In doing so, a different set of priorities may emerge; one that may elicit a higher level of enthusiasm and motivation from the children concerned, especially if they have already received years of clinical treatment.

Rustin and Kuhr (1999, p. 40) also refer to the fundamental distinction between the two models, where problems are seen as deficits of competency (educational model), as opposed to abnormalities of illness (medical model). 'By defining clients' problems as skill deficits and presenting the tools to correct these deficits, the therapist encourages clients to take charge not only of their own treatment but also of some aspects of their own lives as well.'

Rustin and Kuhr continue: 'Learning takes place on different levels: behaviour (specific actions), skills and capabilities (what can be done), beliefs and values (what are the things that matter) and to a lesser degree on the level of identity (basic sense of self, core values)' (p. 41).

Although the notion of the communicatively-impaired child being 'educated' rather than 'treated' may seem controversial, we need to question once again what it is that we as therapists are seeking to do in therapy.

The role of self-esteem and self-efficacy in communication

The previous section of this chapter outlined why it is necessary to adopt a broader understanding of communication, if persistent communication difficulties are to be managed in a holistic way. In building up the conceptual framework of the holistic paradigm being promoted, it is now helpful to highlight the particular relevance to the model of the psychological concepts of self-esteem and self-perception (or self-concept). When these two concepts are added to the framework, it becomes evident that optimal management of persistent difficulties needs to start by returning to fundamentals, that is, how children perceive themselves, since this could hold the key to subsequent successes and failures in therapy. For example, no matter how many resources and how many hours of input clinicians may provide, if children fundamentally believe that they are incapable of achieving what is asked, or that they are fundamentally unworthy and therefore, not worth communicating with, the outcome of therapy may well be disappointing to all concerned. If a child's self-esteem and self-perception are poor, motivation will also be low. In this respect, Dockrell and Messer (1999, p. 151) indicate:

'An important addition to understanding a child's communicative competence is to under-

stand the child's learning history and the implications this may have for the approach taken to tasks. When children believe they can tackle a task, they will learn, given time and appropriate educational opportunities.'

It could be argued that children are motivated to learn when certain fundamental needs are met, that is, when they are not distracted by (among other things):

- physical needs – e.g. physical discomfort (pain/illness, and implications of poverty – hunger, cold, etc.)
- emotional needs – e.g. negative or overwhelming emotions (anxiety, anger, hurt, sadness). Key influences here are whether the home is punitive or nurturing, and the parental/caregiver's attitude towards intervention
- psychosocial needs – e.g. low self-esteem, low self-confidence, poor self-perception and dysfunctional relationships with peers
- communication needs – e.g. difficulties with self-expression hamper socialisation.

These concepts can enhance our understanding as to why a child's progress in speech and language therapy may have plateaued, as well as giving us some valuable insights into how progress might be maintained. For a child who is distracted by any or indeed all of the above needs, the motivation to learn and participate in therapy and in the school classroom, will be adversely affected to some extent.

There is growing awareness of the role mental health plays in a wide range of developmental issues, including learning. For example, a new report notes:

'Another shift in recent public and political perception is that children's mental health is not just a health issue; it is an important educational one as well. It is increasingly acknowledged that a child's state of mind and self-perception have a significant impact on the willingness and ability to concentrate and to learn' (Sylva, 1994). (Hartley-Brewer, 2001, p. 5).

In developing these ideas, we first turn our attention to examining how self-esteem and self-perception develop, and subsequently discuss the relevance of these concepts for managing children with persistant communication deficits.

Development of self-esteem and self-perception

Brumfitt and Sheeran (1999, p. 2) offer clarification of terminology concerned with a child's sense of self, which is often used ambiguously. Part of the reason for this is the continuing lack of consensus on how children think and feel about themselves. Self-concept (or self-perception) can be defined as the sum of all the thoughts and feelings one has about oneself (Rosenberg, 1979). Self-esteem (or self-worth) on the other hand, alludes to the part of the self-concept concerned with evaluating aspects of one's life, such as physical appearance, friendships, thoughts and feelings. It can be described as the 'way that people judge themselves in positive or negative terms'. (p. 2). Dweck (1999, p. 128) advocates a practical explanation:'. . . self-esteem is not a thing that you have or don't have. It is a way of experiencing yourself when you are using your resources well – to master challenges, to learn, to help others.'

Some authorities, however, argue that it is too simplistic to try to differentiate between self-esteem and self-concept since the affective and cognitive domains are so inextricably linked (Damon and Hart, 1988). It is interesting to note that the majority of measures have not successfully discriminated between the two dimensions (Hattie, 1992).

According to Lewis (1990), one of the individual's most significant developmental achievements is to develop a sense of self, by means of acquiring a self-schemata, or set of beliefs about oneself. This is a gradual process that continues through middle childhood and indeed throughout life. Durkin (1995, p. 295) refers to the development of the self-concept (or self-perception) as a 'multifaceted social cognitive process', which is an 'inherently social activity'. He continues:

'Children are engaged in interactions with more mature beings who are very interested in them, and who provide both context and guidance. We need other people in order to determine what is distinctive about our own self.

. . . does mean that we are affected by other people's emphases on social and psychological properties, and by their expectations about who we should become.'

In identifying the development of self-esteem, several psychologists (including Erikson, 1963) have highlighted the significance of a child's early affective or emotional experiences (especially with a primary caregiver). As infants detect friendly or hostile environments, and acceptance or disapproval from significant others, they gradually develop a fundamental sense of content or discontent, and pride or shame from early social interactions. It is in their everyday interactions with other people (notably parents) that pre-schoolers accumulate and store feedback on the appropriateness of their behaviour, language and ideas. The extent to which they receive approval or disapproval is thought to play an important role in the development of the self. Elkind (for example, 1988) underlines the importance of the quality of the relationship between a child and significant others in the development of high self-esteem. Where the relationship is strong and rewarding, self-esteem is more likely to flourish.

Bandura (1986) suggests that self-definition also arises from a child's sense of self-efficacy, which stems from growing confidence in influencing the environment. Bandura (1997, p. 11) distinguishes between perceived self-efficacy and self-esteem, the former derives from judgements about personal capability, whereas the latter is rooted in judgements about self-worth. Further attention will be paid to the role of self-efficacy later in this chapter.

Rosenberg (1986) proposes that this evolving perception of worthiness is probably not only the basis of self-esteem in childhood, but also influences adult self-perception and outlook on life later on (Pelham and Swann, 1989, p. 672). In summarising the research evidence, Pelham and Swann (1989, p. 677) indicate '. . . it appears that people's general sense of self-worth is determined by three distinct factors: (a) their positive and negative feelings about themselves, (b) their specific beliefs about themselves, and (c) the way that they frame these beliefs'. These factors may be a combination of independent affective and cognitive components.

However, as Cairns and Cairns (1988) point out, developing a sense of identity is not purely a cognitive task, because we attach values and salience to ourselves. As will become evident in the later discussion of coping, it appears that high self-esteem may enhance children's resilience in coping with stress (Ruble and Thompson, 1992). Mruk (1999, p. 92) also endorses the advantages of high self-esteem:

'Factors associated with positive self-esteem . . . such as increased autonomy, greater openness to alternatives, and a higher confidence in one's perceptions and abilities, all predispose one toward favorable outcomes in dealing with problems, challenges, and opportunities, in general.'

In mapping developmental trends, Harter (1988) notes that the self-concepts of pre-school children generally show little negativity or organisation, as they have not yet developed a global notion of self-worth. Instead, they appear to base their self-judgements on specific domains. This tendency is evident in their usually positive self-descriptions which comprise disjointed features, concerning their possessions, achievements and personal characteristics.

The pervasively positive attitude displayed by pre-schoolers, however, changes with age as children become increasingly conscious of their uniqueness and of other evaluations and expectations of them. This is apparent in middle childhood when children's self-definitions usually include evaluative statements (or self-affects), and assessments of their own competence, both of which are influenced by socialising with others. Self-descriptions at this stage tend to reflect a combination of pride in certain areas of achievement and attributes and shame or inadequacy in others (Harter, 1983, 1988).

A global concept of self-worth (or self-esteem) is evident from around the age of 8, when children have sufficient emotional and cognitive maturity to integrate information about different aspects of their lives (Marsh et al., 1991). Harter (1987) notes that an important relationship exists between self-perception and self-esteem. In her study, she asked children to rate themselves according to five areas (social

competence, scholastic competence, athletic competence, physical appearance and behavioural conduct), and on general self-esteem. The findings suggest that where children detect a discrepancy between their competence and the significance they attach to that competence, their own global self-esteem tended to suffer. This outcome can help in understanding how the self-esteem and self-perception of communicatively-impaired children interact, to result in diminished self-confidence, especially regarding the important act of communicating (Durkin, 1995, p. 300).

Experiences related to school can influence the individual's evolving self-concept, since evidence suggests that during the early years of schooling self-esteem can diminish (Ruble, 1994). 'Initially optimistic appraisals of one's capacities and prospects tend to be challenged by discoveries of one's limitations, by the experiences of setbacks and difficulties in new educational tasks, and by social comparisons with peers who may be ahead in some domains (for example, Marsh, 1985)' (Durkin, 1995, p. 301).

Marsh (1985) notes that as the optimistic self-concepts of pre-schoolers may be unrealistic, this lowering of self-esteem is not necessarily an adverse development.

Relevance of self-esteem and self-perception for understanding a child's experience of living with impaired communication on a daily basis

Having outlined the development of self-esteem and self-concept in childhood, we now turn our attention to their relevance for understanding a child's experience of living with dysfunctional communication on a daily basis. An important starting point is to remember the significance of peers on reaching school, since comparison with peers becomes an increasingly critical aspect of a child's experience at this age. Various authorities note the influence peers can exert on the psychosocial development of young people. For example, Frydenberg (1997, p. 75) points out:

'How we view ourselves is closely linked to our successes and failures, how others view us and how we compare ourselves to others. Self-concept . . . is an important factor in determining behaviour.'

Brumfitt and Sheeran (1999, p. 2) identify social feedback and social comparisons as two of the most eminent influences on self-esteem at any given time (Festinger, 1954). Social feedback denotes information about ourselves which we receive from those around us. It can be either verbal (for instance, praise or compliments) or non-verbal (for example, others seeking out our company). Social comparisons, on the other hand, allude to the comparisons we tend to make between ourselves and others. Although self-esteem is considered to be a relatively stable characteristic over time (a trait), the nature of the feedback we receive and the social comparisons made can determine how positively or negatively we see ourselves at any given moment.

In taking account of feedback and interpersonal comparisons, we seem to evaluate their potency for us according to how close we feel to the person making the comments. For example, if we do not know the person well our self-esteem and self-concept are not likely to be as affected by the feedback as if the person concerned was our best friend. Likewise, the aspect of the self-concept being compared to others must be of significance to us if it is to influence our self-esteem (Brumfitt and Sheeran, 1999, p. 3).

Relevance of self-esteem and self-perception for speech and language therapy

In considering the management of persistent communication difficulties, we need now to ask ourselves again, what relevance do the theoretical concepts of self-esteem and self-concept (or self-perception) have for effective speech and language therapy? For the answer to this question, we will identify first what helps children to thrive in psychosocial terms. That is, what is most likely to nurture their self-esteem and so enhance their self-perception? By taking such findings on board, we can incorporate them into our clinical work, and be assured that we have created the most appropriate therapeutic relationship and conducive environment for optimal learning during therapy.

We know already from various literatures that children thrive when they:

- receive approval from a significant adult (parent, schoolteacher, speech and language therapist)
- sense that they can do what is asked of them
- feel knowledge is worth acquiring
- feel that their efforts are recognised if not rewarded
- feel safe
- are not distracted by anxieties.

All of these (and many more, since this list is not exhaustive) point to the fundamental significance of children feeling good about themselves in order to thrive during the pre-school years and in order to continue to thrive on reaching the challenging task of school. It becomes apparent, in identifying what makes children thrive, that all the factors listed above directly affect motivation. If motivation is low or even lacking altogether, children are unlikely to progress satisfactorily. Thus, in order to equip a communicatively-impaired child with a psychological survival kit, we need to pay attention to what we already know about child-rearing and then translate its relevance for therapy. As Mruk (1999, p. 82) highlights: '. . . it is competence at meeting the challenges of life that is especially relevant to self-esteem, and not merely being successful or doing something effectively.'

If we now consider the additional challenges for children with impaired communication, it becomes obvious that before we can expect any success in our prescribed objectives (focused on aspects such as articulation, phonology and language development), we need to spend time first building up these children's positive feelings about themselves.

Within the field of health psychology, there is growing awareness of the need to incorporate attention to patients' psychosocial needs into their clinical management. For example, Davis and Fallowfield (1991) allude to the general neglect of patients' psychosocial difficulties with the overemphasis on the medical model:

'Perversely, as our ability to treat disease and disability increases, many more individuals face a lifetime of chronic handicap or ill-health. Providing them with the sorts of psychological support and encouraging coping strategies likely to maximise and enhance their quality of life is a vital part of care' (Preface, p.xi).

The key terms here are 'psychological support' and 'encouraging coping strategies', since they are directly associated with nurturing self-esteem and an individual's perception that he or she does have the personal resources to cope. Other authorities refer to these capabilities as 'social competence'. For instance, Kapp-Simon and McGuire (1997, p. 380) note that 'In recent years, there has been increasing recognition of the importance of social competence as a component of psychological health (e.g. Dodge et al., 1986)'.

Putallaz and Gottman (1981) define social competence as: 'aspects of social behavior that are important with respect to preventing physical illness or psychopathology in children and adults'. Thus, social interaction between peers can influence the emergence of social competence. The authors go on to describe the socially competent individual as: '. . . one who is able to generate a response to an interpersonal situation that is appropriate and meets the demands of that situation.' (Kapp-Simon and McGuire, 1997, p. 380).

The particular relevance of enhancing a child's social competence for speech and language therapy, can be seen in understanding that speech is a vital vehicle for social interaction and peer group membership. Where a child's social interactions are hampered by dysfunctional communication, there is an almost predictable cascade of associated psychosocial difficulties with which he or she will have to contend:

'A child with previous peer failures may feel less competent socially and, as a result approach social interaction so tentatively as to make success almost impossible (Rubin and Stewart, 1996).' (Kapp-Simon and McGuire, 1997, p. 383).

Rustin and Kuhr (1999, p. 81) offer insight into the classroom experiences of the socially ineffective child. In particular, they note the tendency for such a child to be on the periphery of the 'social system' within the class, and to be perceived as passive or isolated rather than actively engaged in group activities. When attempting to interact with peers, a socially inept child may be rejected by peers. In this way, schooling may reinforce the child's sense of inadequacy, which in turn may profoundly affect a child's motivation to learn unless they are helped to overcome such fundamental obstacles. Dockrell and Messer (1999, p. 59) endorse this finding in the context of 'disabled' children:

'The majority of studies show that there are significant differences between the status of 'disabled' and 'non-disabled' students in mainstream classrooms. Studies of children with general delays, specific learning difficulties, specific language impairments, hearing impairments and physical disabilities have all shown that these students experience peer rejection (Horne, 1985).'

Having considered the relevance of the psychological concepts of self-esteem, self-efficacy and social competence for effective management of persistent communication difficulties, we now turn our attention to their longer-term consequences for the child.

Victimisation, ostracisation and stigmatisation: identifying the VOS cycle of disadvantage

The previous section looked at the concepts of self-esteem and social competence in the context of dysfunctional communication. This section now examines the consequences of having high or low self-esteem (positive or negative psychosocial status) and the relationship between self-esteem and coping with adversity. A model is proposed in the form of a matrix, which shows possible relationships between dysfunctional communication and psychosocial status. In the course of discussing the implications of the matrix, it will become apparent that there is a group of children who are particularly at risk for experiencing the cycle of consequences that tend to emanate from having a negative psychosocial status. In the light of this, we will argue that there is a pressing need to incorporate the wider implications of dysfunctional communication into the clinical management of persisting speech and language problems.

The relationship between how we feel and think about ourselves, and how we cope with the challenges we encounter in everyday life, is arguably a very close and intricate one. For example, if we feel good about ourselves, we are far more likely to be able to cope with difficult situations, than if we feel inadequate and helpless as individuals. The matrix in Figure 2.1 (derived from Mruk, 1999) is one means of exploring the relationship between psychosocial functioning (and ability to cope with adversity) and dysfunctional communication. It is divided into four quadrants or domains. On the vertical axis is the continuum negative–positive psychosocial status (self-esteem, self-perception, motivation to achieve, coping style). The horizontal axis represents the continuum of dysfunctional–competent

communication. Each of the quadrants will be now introduced in outlining the implications of each for the individuals concerned.

Heatherton and Ambady (1993) among others, refer to one's general coping 'style'. Roger (1997, p. 73), however, asserts that there are 'maladaptive' and 'adaptive' coping styles. In this context, the term 'style' refers to our habitual way of responding to challenging and difficult situations. Thus, according to Roger: 'Maladaptive styles have the effect of making us more vulnerable while adaptive styles help us to deal with demands'. The implications of the differing styles will become apparent in discussing each of the four groupings of the matrix in Figure 2.1, before considering the role of coping strategies in managing persistent communication difficulties.

Matrix to show possible relationships between dysfunctional communication and psychosocial status

Positive Psychosocial Status
(eg high self esteem, positive self-perception, adaptive coping style, therefore, high motivation to achieve)

Adaptive-dysfunctional:
- Positive self-esteem
- Positive self-perception
- Social competence hampered by dysfunctional communication
- Sense of self-efficacy
- Adaptive coping style

The 'resilient copers'

Adaptive-competent:
- Positive self-esteem
- Positive self-perception
- Socially competent
- Sense of self-efficacy
- Adaptive coping style

The non-impaired norm

Dysfunctional Communication | *Competent Communication*

Maladaptive dysfunctional:
- Disadvantaged by negative self-esteem
- Disadvantaged by negative self-perception
- Socially incompetent due to constellation of disadvantages
- Little sense of self-efficacy
- Maladaptive coping style

The 'at risk' group

Maladaptive-competent:
- Negative self-esteem
- Negative self-perception
- Potential to be socially competent but lacks confidence
- Little sense of self-efficacy
- Maladaptive coping style

The hampered competent

Negative Psychosocial Status
(eg low self-esteem, poor self-perception, maladaptive coping style, therefore, low motivation to achieve)

Figure 2.1 Matrix to show possible relationships between dysfunctional communication and psychosocial status.

1. Adaptive-competent – represents the non-impaired, well-functioning 'norm'

Key characteristics:

- positive self-esteem
- positive perception of self
- socially competent
- sense of self-efficacy
- adaptive coping style

Adaptive-competent individuals are those without persistent communication difficulties, who are effective communicators with a positive sense of self and their capabilities. In this context, they are included to denote the 'norm', where positive psychosocial status and competent communication together combine to produce an upward spiral of rewarding relationships with peers, optimal learning at school and a sense of self-efficacy.

2. Adaptive-dysfunctional – the 'resilient copers'

Key characteristics:

- positive self-esteem
- positive perception of self
- social competence hampered by dysfunctional communication
- sense of self-efficacy
- adaptive coping style

There appears to be a group of children with dysfunctional communication, who may have severe difficulties, yet are able to cope in a remarkable way with their evident disabilities. It seems that they are driven by positive feelings about their capabilities and self-worth, and a strong sense of who they are. In addition, they often have a keen sense of humour and a positive outlook on life. Unlike their disadvantaged contemporaries they feel that they can cope in challenging situations. Rutter (1985) identifies three elements that characterise resilience:

'Firstly, a sense of self-esteem and confidence; secondly a belief in one's own self-efficacy and ability to deal with change and adaptation;

and thirdly, a repertoire of social problem solving approaches.'

The irony is, of course, that resilient children are less likely to be picked on and bullied, because peers sense their resilience. That is, they are not perceived to be 'soft and easy' targets.

Resilience has also been identified as a key element of mental health alongside positive self-esteem. For example, Holland (2000) describes mental health as: 'the emotional and spiritual resilience that enables us to enjoy life and to survive pain, suffering and disappointment. It is a positive sense of well-being and an underlying belief in our own worth and the worth of others.' Holland also acknowledges that the way in which we communicate, think and feel directly affects the nature of our interactions, experiences and responses.

Taylor and Brown (1988) have identified several optimistic dispositions which mentally healthy and happy people appear to employ in maintaining a positive psychological state. One example of this is the tendency to overestimate one's capabilities and talents. Pelham and Swann (1989, p. 678) however, found that:

'… people might bolster their self-esteem in a manner that requires no distortion whatsoever – that is, by framing their specific self-views in a manner that is favorable to themselves. Thus, although the proverbial 98-lb weakling might be unable to convince others that he is the next Mr. Olympia, he is completely free to decide that an Olympian physique is of little importance to him. In this way, he may concede his wimpiness without experiencing any damage to his self-esteem.'

Other authorities have highlighted the role of protective factors which some children possess, and examine why and what it is that enables some children to be resilient copers, whereas others clearly suffer the consequences of disadvantage. Luthar et al. (2000, p. 543) describe resilience as: 'a dynamic process encompassing positive adaptation within the context of significant adversity.' They note that resilience research can greatly enhance understanding of the processes affecting individuals who are vulnerable and at risk. In discussing protective factors, Rutter and Rutter (1993, p. 55) refer to the 'role of catalytic mechanisms that either enhance resistance to risk factors (protection) or reduce it (vulnerability)'. Self-esteem and self-efficacy are identified as key mediating mechanisms. The use of effective coping strategies, general cognitive ability and personality variables may also be significant protective factors. The question of causality in understanding the part played by the catalytic mechanisms is of particular interest, as it has implications for potential therapeutic interventions.

As Nash (1995, p. 210) reports, various efforts have been made to identify the essence of resilience coping, especially in the context of bullying:

'. . . it appears that an ability to deflect the potentially injurious teasing comments is especially significant. Kobasa (1979) has advanced the useful concept of "hardiness", to describe the resilience with which some individuals are able to cope with adverse situations. This notion implicates a sense of psychological "detachment" (Roger, 1992) from the incident while it is happening, and as such is identified as an integral component of adaptive "coping style".'

That is, a key part of the deflection is not internalising the pernicious comments. Although this ability appears to come naturally to some youngsters, it can also be learned as a coping strategy by others, as will become evident in discussing the activities related to handling bullying (Chapter 3).

Having identified that some children are 'resilient copers' in the face of adversity, the pressing question is how and why only a proportion of youngsters possess this vital advantage. Frydenberg (1997, p. 80) asks the challenging question: 'What is it that makes the difference?' Clearly, temperament and factors associated with maturation play their part in developing effective coping strategies, but is there something more than the simple passing of time or one's family background that accounts for this difference? She continues:

'What a person does impacts on their environment, outcomes in turn impact on the chain of events that are associated with coping. What one does, and how it is received, in turn affects how one feels about oneself and how an

individual responds on future occasions. Opportunities to reflect on coping enable individuals to take charge of their actions rather than be passive respondents.' (p. 80).

Resilient copers will be discussed again when we look at the role of coping mechanisms.

3. Maladaptive-competent – those who have the potential but are hampered in some way

Key characteristics:

- negative self-esteem
- negative perception of self
- potential to be socially competent but lacks confidence
- little sense of self-efficacy
- maladaptive coping style

As Figure 2.1 shows, these individuals have the potential to be effective and competent communicators, but are hampered by low self-esteem and a poor perception of themselves. Whereas the two 'adaptive' groups already discussed seem to encounter the consequences of an 'upward' spiral of positive experiences, the two 'maladaptive' groups appear to experience the converse. Although the majority of communicatively-impaired children and adolescents learn how to cope with challenging situations during their school years, the vulnerable minority learn helplessness (Seligman, 1975). Hopson and Scally (1981, e.g. p. 53) suggest that individuals can either learn self-empowerment or become 'depowered'. By identifying the vulnerable minority, those who are depowered can be helped to become self-empowered (Nash, 1995), and this is one of the primary objectives of the programme being promoted.

4. Maladaptive-dysfunctional – 'at risk' group for psychosocial dysfunction

Key characteristics:

- disadvantaged by negative self-esteem
- disadvantaged by negative perception of self

- socially incompetent due to constellation of disadvantages
- little sense of self-efficacy
- maladaptive coping style

To gain an insight into the experiences of this group, try to imagine what it must be like to live with impaired communication on a daily basis, as a school child. As a child with a long-term communication difficulty, you know that you sound different from other people. You may also look different, too (for example, cleft lip and palate or cerebral palsy). Every time you go to school, you know that someone may pick on you and call you nasty names or push you around. You know it's no good answering back, because whatever you say is mimicked. You may even be teased by your own teacher, or a member of your family. Sometimes, you are so afraid of being picked on that you don't say anything in class and you stay near the teacher at playtime. You may feel that because you are different nobody wants to be your friend. When you go home, you may not even tell anyone what horrible things have been said or done to you; you prefer to lock them up inside and try to be brave (Nash, 1997).

What has this got to do with communication? The answer is 'everything', since communication is the means by which we enjoy social and personal relationships with others (or not as the case may be). Indeed, it is precisely because communication requires interacting with and relating to others, that it should be seen as something which involves the total person, and not just the acquisition of adequate

speech and language. How can such needs be effectively addressed?

Within the cleft population, which typifies many problems associated with persistent communication dysfunction, there is sufficient evidence to suggest that long-term communication difficulties may be indicative of wider psychosocial problems (such as social isolation, and poor coping strategies). That is, dysfunctional communication may be only one factor in a constellation of factors that militates against the individual's personal and social competence. We are now keen to broaden the scope of the current study to include other client groups with persisting communication difficulties, to investigate this area further.

Children with persistent communication problems could be at risk for developing the VOS cycle of disadvantage, whereby a child is victimised, ostracised and stigmatised, notably by peers in and outside school, as indicated in Figure 2.2 (Nash et al., 2001b). These three terms describe different forms of abusive behaviour. The Concise Oxford Dictionary offers the following definitions:

- **victimise** – to 'single out for punishment or unfair treatment'
- **ostracise** – to 'exclude (a person) from a society ... refuse to associate with'
- **stigmatise** – to 'describe as unworthy or disgraceful' (from Greek 'to mark with a brand').

These behaviours collectively suggest problems with peer relationships, which are a critical determinant of a child's experience of school.

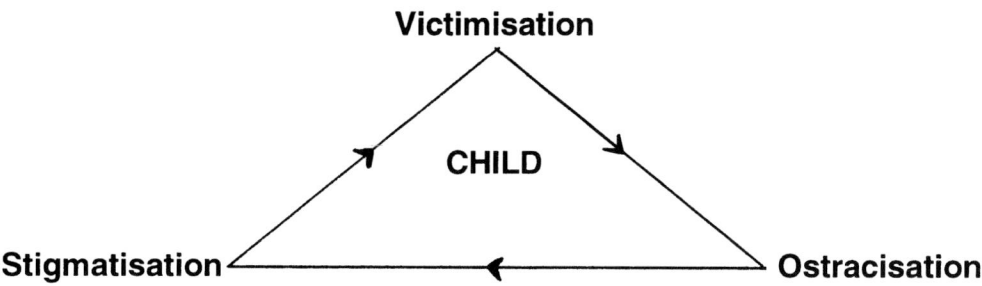

Figure 2.2 The VOS cycle of disadvantage.

A child who is caught up in the VOS cycle of disadvantage may experience a variety of 'knock-on' effects, not least a sense of loneliness, helplessness, hopelessness and bewilderment. This predicament is made all the more painful by the growing developmental importance attached to what peers think, as Erwin (1993, p. 215) highlights:

'As peers become increasingly significant in the lives of children and adolescents, satisfaction with peer relationships becomes increasingly important as a determinant of loneliness and the influence of parents declines (Schultz and Moore, 1989).'

This assertion endorses the outcome of Parker and Asher's (1987, p. 357) literature review, which generally supports the hypothesis that problematic peer relationships in childhood are a risk factor for difficulties in later life.

Erwin (1993, p. 216) describes a complex network of social factors which are associated with loneliness and which implicate various cognitive and social skills deficits (such as poor self-perception and low self-esteem). In combination, these factors provide the foundation for a self-fulfilling prophecy, in which loneliness becomes self-perpetuating into adolescence and beyond (Hymel and Franke, 1985). It is also these very factors that make a child susceptible to bullying, since bullies tend to seek out those whom they perceive to be vulnerable, especially those with some form of disability (for example, Smith, 1999). In doing so, they effectively push their victim into the VOS cycle of disadvantage. Therefore, enhancing the victim's social competence may conceivably make them less attractive to bullies and less of an easy target.

Clinicians and teachers can play a significant role by taking note of the 'danger' signs as they occur, in order to identify the most vulnerable children. It is precisely because long-term communication problems in themselves do not warrant the attentions of a clinical psychologist that the broader psychosocial difficulties, of which communication problems are a part, may be passed over or even ignored altogether. Having said this, educational psychologists may be involved in combating bullying problems in schools, but they may not have direct involvement

with communicatively-impaired children unless those concerned have special educational needs.

Unless the wider psychosocial aspects of dysfunctional communication are addressed, there may be indications of psychopathology in the individuals concerned (such as depression or even suicide). Indeed, Mruk (1999, p. 165) notes that poor self-esteem is implicated in various diagnosable mental health problems. Because of this association, he comments that professional help is often needed for those with serious self-esteem problems. Asher and Coie (1990) underline the relationship between peer rejection (and peer isolation) and the notably increased risk for various psychosocial and psychiatric problems in later life. The possible consequences of unresolved persisting communication difficulties are shown in Figure 2.3.

Goodyer (2000) points out that the adverse experience of living with impaired communication may place an individual at risk for antisocial or emotional problems. Over the past 30 years it has emerged that approximately 50% of children with speech and language impairment show a range of related emotional and behavioural difficulties. This rate is over three times that for the general community (for example, Beitchman et al., 1990). Goodyer continues (2000, p. 228):

'For some young children these associated difficulties appear to be an understandable consequence of their speech and language impairment, such as persistent frustration at failing to make their needs and desires understood.'

Mruk (1999, p. 95) further suggests a link between self-esteem and psychopathology:

'One way that self-esteem and depression seem to be connected is that, insofar as self-esteem protects the individual against setbacks, cracks in this shield allow depression to take hold more easily. The individual then becomes more vulnerable to stressors. Increased vulnerability means less capacity for problem solving and coping effectively, which leads to an erosion of worthiness and hope. The resulting sense of hopelessness is understood as a strong risk for suicide (Durand and Barlow, 1997). In this sense, we can see self-esteem as a life-and-death issue.'

A recent report, produced by the Department for Education and Skills (2001, p. 6)

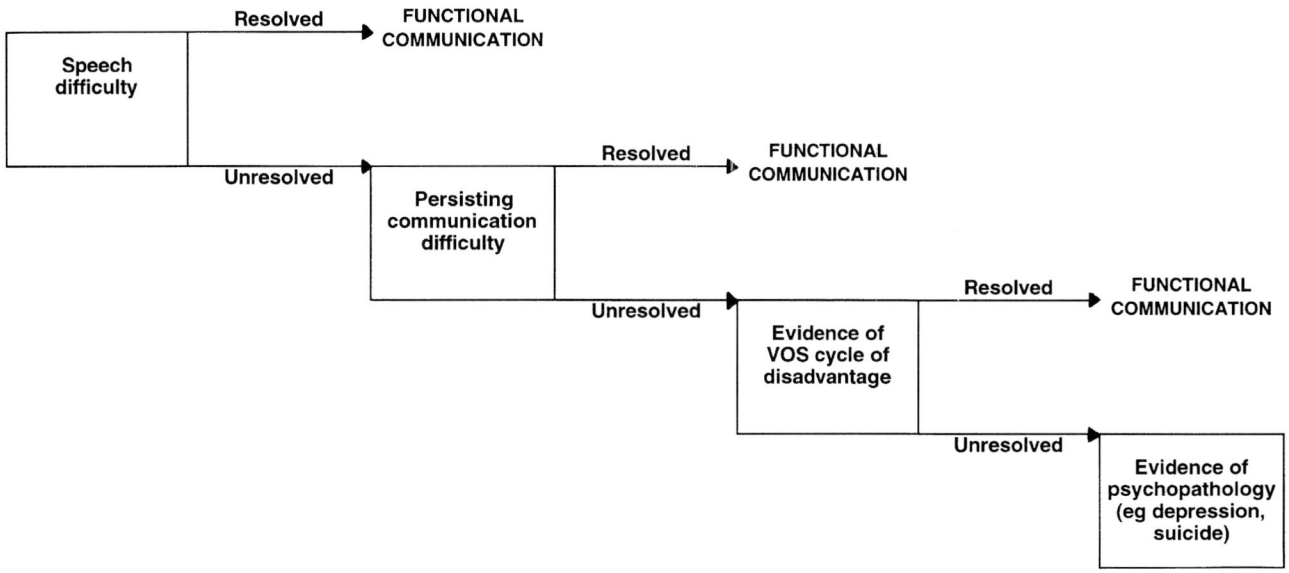

Figure 2.3 Possible consequences of unresolved persistent communication difficulties (or chronic communication dysfunction).

on promoting children's mental health, asserts that risk factors are cumulative. That is, as they increase, more protective factors are required to counterbalance them: '. . . when risk factors and stressful life events outweigh the protective factors, even the most resilient individual can develop problems.'

Although the association between poor self-esteem and depression is well documented, the cause and effect relationship that exists between them is still unclear. Brumfitt and Sheeran (1999, p. 4) refer to the ongoing debate as to whether floundering self-esteem causes depression, or poor self-esteem is a consequence of depression. The bulk of evidence appears to suggest that low self-esteem comes first but this is still controversial, and it is possible that self-esteem and depression influence each other. Mruk (1999, p. 95) endorses this view by indicating that once a pattern emerges, difficulties with low self-esteem and depression are both more probable and more severe. This relationship is evident in various clinical studies (for example, Tennen and Affleck, 1993).

Poor self-esteem has also been linked to certain types of juvenile delinquency by Kaplan et al. (1986). One explanation for this is that adoles-

cents (in particular) generally attempt to achieve a modicum of self-esteem, by seeking peer acceptance and demonstrating success in some valued domain (such as sport). However, when these socially acceptable ways of gaining high self-esteem are denied to them, for whatever reason, young people turn to other, less socially acceptable alternatives to bolster their self-esteem.

The role of coping strategies – why are some children so resilient?

By unravelling the implications of the four groupings shown in the matrix above (Figure 2.1), it seems that in terms of social competence (which lies at the heart of effective communication), it may be possible to 'plot' the groupings on a continuum (Figure 2.4). It is apparent from the figure that it is the coping style (adaptive or maladaptive), rather than the state of the individual's communication capabilities (dysfunctional or competent), that determines the position on the continuum. That is, on closer inspection, the continuum indicates the importance of effective and adaptive coping strategies, since it appears to be the ability or inability to cope with communication difficulties on a daily

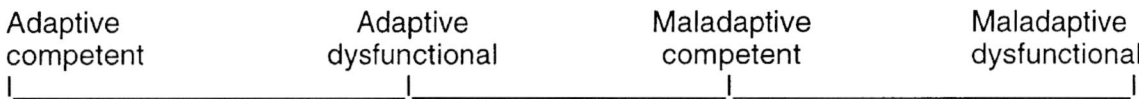

| Adaptive competent | Adaptive dysfunctional | Maladaptive competent | Maladaptive dysfunctional |

Figure 2.4 Continuum suggesting degrees of social competence.

basis that is the essential determinant of whether a child ultimately 'sinks' or 'swims' when speech and language therapy has ceased, or when speech and language progress plateaus in spite of continued intervention.

It is useful to remind ourselves at this point, what it is that the communicatively-impaired child has to cope with. With reference to the matrix, for children in the 'maladaptive-dysfunctional' quadrant, the answer is potentially a great deal. For example, they may have to cope with any or all of the potential stressors (that is, something which evidently causes stress) shown in Table 2.1. Expressed this way, it is evident that communication impairment can be a very real and persistent stressor for these children, in addition to other more readily identifiable stressors, such as bullying in the playground or being excluded by peers. It can be a revealing and useful exercise in understanding a child's

response to therapy and school to identify all the compounding pressures with which they are expected to cope on a daily basis.

As stated earlier, it is impossible to predict the outcome for children with persistent communication difficulties, since the longer the impairment continues the more likely it is that the difficulty will accumulate other psychosocial difficulties in its wake. Indeed, it could be argued that although it is essential to offer therapy to those with long-term communication difficulties, perhaps the therapist should be realistic in the assessment of just how much can be achieved, given the time pressures of a heavy caseload. It is precisely for this reason that equipping a child with a psychosocial 'survival kit' of coping strategies needs to be incorporated into the clinical management of persistent communication problems. This should in no way be seen as compromising the best efforts of the therapist to

Table 2.1 Characteristics and consequences of persistent communication difficulties

Characteristics

Degree of speech impairment

Inadequate social skills (such as turn-taking, eye contact)

Poor listening skills

Insufficient repair strategies (what to do when communication breaks down)

Tension (physical and mental) which can produce vocal abuse

Possible language impairment (poor understanding and inability to express feelings, thoughts and ideas in words)

Consequences
The child may experience:

Poor self-esteem and poor self-perception

Poor social and personal relationships largely due to inadequate social skills

Indications of social inadequacy: (VOS cycle)

Social withdrawal and downward spiral of negative experiences with consequent adverse effect on schooling and learning

Educational problems, such as difficulties with literacy and numeracy

Poor health, such as stress-related illness and possible psychopathology (e.g. depression)

resolve the dysfunctional communication problem completely, nor should attention to coping strategies be seen as a second-best alternative. Rather, it is offering these children a very real and valuable means of coping with their impairment for life.

Implications of coping strategies for managing persistent communication difficulties

Management of school-aged children with persisting communication difficulties needs to be seen as something distinct from management of pre-school children, whose communication problems are expected to resolve by the age of school entry. This distinction may be evident in the aims and objectives of the therapists concerned. For example, whereas pre-school children (and parents or caregivers) may be well motivated to work with a therapist on clearly defined objectives, often for a specified period of time, it is important for everyone involved in managing school-aged children to be aware that they (and their parents or caregivers) may find the same framework of therapy demotivating and disheartening if it continues once schooling has begun. It may also be disruptive to school attendance. Thus, a different emphasis and different experience of therapy may be required to enable a child to move forwards (rather than regress, as sometimes happens).

In view of the four groupings of the matrix (Figure 2.1), we need to ask why and what it is that enables some children to be resilient copers, whereas others clearly suffer the consequences of disadvantage. One factor that might account for this apparent difference is the nature of a child's self-talk; that is, the type of self-instruction children give themselves that reinforces the positive or indeed negative feelings they have about themselves. In this way, the type of self-talk may be largely determined by the state of the child's self-esteem. In turn, the self-talk reflects and endorses the child's perception of themselves. Nash (1998, p. 62) describes the nature of self-talk in which we all engage throughout the day:

'Inside my head there is a continuous patter going on. Often it is the parent in me

urging on the child; or it may be the child protesting at what is being asked of it ... If I listen, I can break into these habitual repetitions and take them in hand. It may be that they could be made more constructive, working for me and others rather than against us.'

Where a child's self-talk is negative and denigrating, it can fuel the realisation of a self-fulfilling prophecy, in which the child's experiences of communicating with others results in unrewarding relationships with peers, social isolation, loneliness, victimisation and so forth in a seemingly unrelenting circle. This can be seen in Figure 2.5, which charts the vicious circle that can arise and which is likely, in part, to be reinforced by the child's habitually negative self-talk (model based on Harter, 1997).

Meichenbaum (1975) developed the cognitive approach of 'self-instructional training', whereby an individual can be helped to change the nature of their self-talk. This is achieved by focusing on more adaptive self-talk and guiding the person away from distressing, maladaptive thoughts. Such instruction can play a key role in moderating the type of self-talk in which children engage and then helping them to learn effective coping strategies, which over time can become habitual responses to difficult situations. The reader is referred to Rustin and Kuhr's useful discussion of how such training can be put into practice for communicatively-impaired children (1999, p. 28).

In attempting to define what characterises 'resilient copers', it could be that they tend not only to have a healthy self-esteem and a robust sense of identity (self-perception), but also that these are fuelled by positive and nurturing self-talk. It is also feasible that these individuals possess an adaptive coping style that serves to buffer them against the damaging effects of stress and anxiety on both mental and physical health, which are well documented in the literature (for example, Sheridan and Radmacher, 1992).

Mruk (1999, p. 92) provides a particularly eloquent explanation of the link between stress and self-esteem:

'Stress can certainly tax our sense of worthiness as a person, especially if it comes from a negative source and is prolonged. The shielding function of self-esteem seems to help to reduce

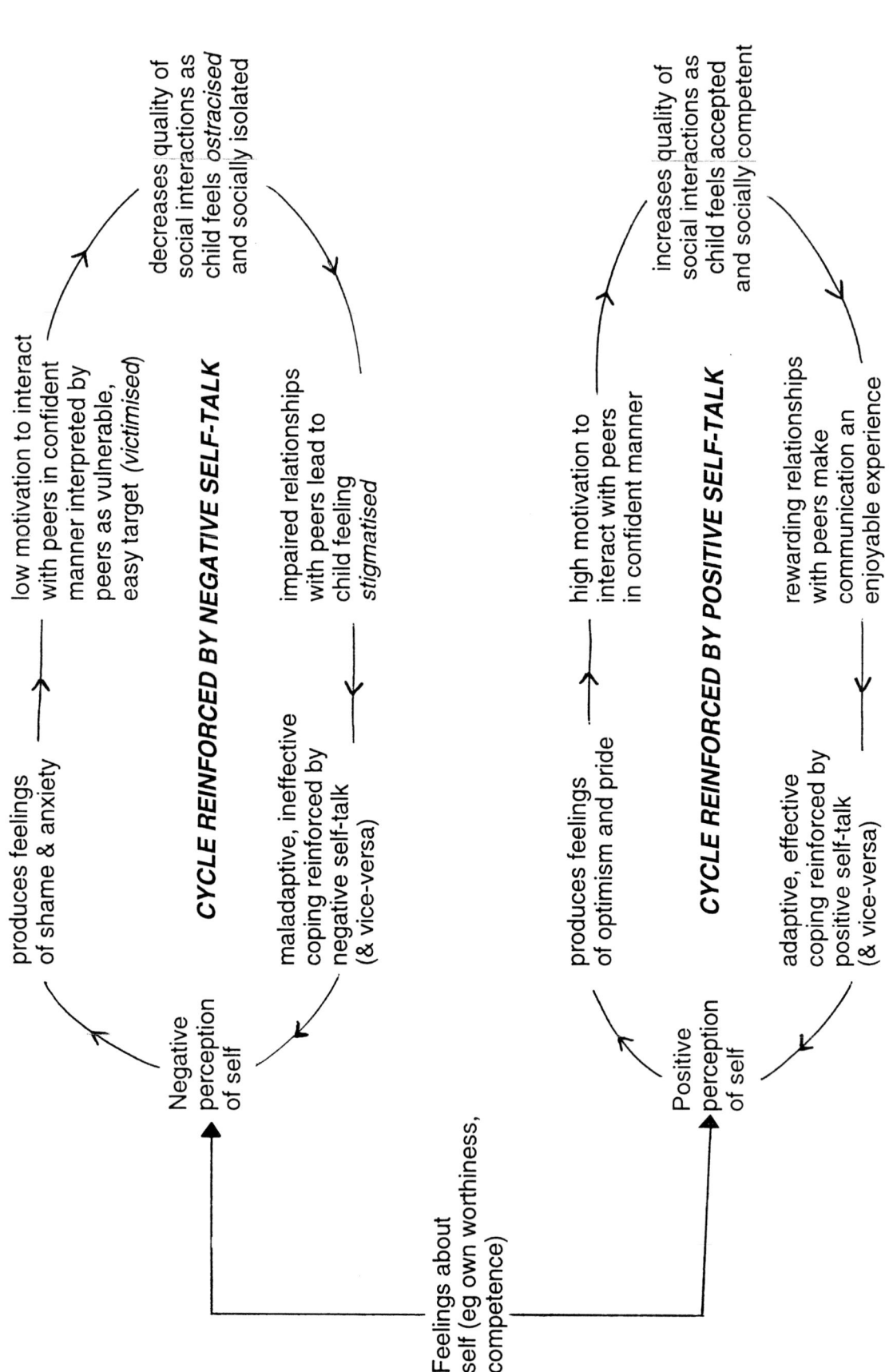

Figure 2.5 How a self-fulfilling prophecy is reinforced by the child's self-talk and turns into a vicious circle (the VOS cycle of disadvantage).

the negative power of stress by providing some insulation for how we feel about ourselves during such a period. The possible negative effects of stress on our perceptions of self and the world, the meanings we give to what is happening to us, and the actions we select in response to a stressful situation are all influenced by how good this shield happens to be. People with high self-esteem are generally at an advantage in this regard because they are better protected from suffering temporary declines of worthiness associated with failure, loss, or rejection.'

Frey and Carlock (1989, p. 107) suggest that the lower the individual's self-esteem, the more likely it is to be disturbed by the mildest of challenges in life, and the more resistant the person's self-esteem becomes to healthy development.

A further characteristic of 'resilient copers' can be gleaned from Seiffge-Krenke's (1990) work which found a relationship between self-concept and coping. In that study, 'active' copers tended to have high self-esteem and enjoyed good relationships with their parents. 'Problem avoiders' on the other hand, offered depressed descriptions of themselves, and were not confident of their own capabilities. In view of this, it is surmised that self-esteem may determine one's choice of coping strategies. In turn, the use of those strategies may help to determine one's self-concept and shape self-esteem. Thus, positive self-esteem is in itself an adaptive and effective coping strategy (Frydenberg, 1997, p. 76).

In a follow-up study of cleft-impaired children, Nash (1995, p. 206) examined whether effective coping mechanisms are a function of innate and/or learned behavioural responses to environmental stimuli. Three groups were identified on the basis of responses to teasing or bullying, as outlined below:

- group 1 – innate or 'natural' resilience, e.g. evident in humouring the bully
- group 2 – learned resilience, e.g. evident in learning to ignore the bully
- group 3 – 'at risk': lacks innate or learned resilience to avert potential injury by the bully.

These groupings suggest that there is a variety of responses to bullying, which may derive from a combination of genetic and environmental factors. Some youngsters appear to be blessed with a natural resilience, whereas others have to learn how to cope effectively. Others still appear to be 'at risk' for psychosocial dysfunction and need further help in mastering adaptive coping strategies.

Having pinpointed some of the essential characteristics of 'resilient copers', we now need to consider what implications this finding has for managing persistent communication problems in clinic. The first question is, how feasible is it to develop these desirable characteristics in others, and is this a valuable use of limited management resources? In responding to the first of these questions, it is enlightening to note Frydenberg's (1997, p. 77) observation regarding whether the focus of intervention should be on enhancing self-esteem or developing effective coping strategies. For a long time the tendency has been on the former, but growing evidence suggests that emphasis on increasing a repertoire of coping skills may be a more productive approach, and one which will lead to improved self-esteem (Seligman, 1995). However, as Roskies and Lazarus (1980, p. 57) note, possessing competent coping strategies is not sufficient, one also needs to believe that one possesses them. In this context, Sarafino (1990, p. 115) points out that a robust sense of self-efficacy is associated with experiencing lower psychological strain in stressful situations, compared with a weaker sense of self-efficacy (for example, Bandura et al., 1985).

The second question concerns the relative value of committing scarce resources to such intervention programmes. One of the major strengths of our residential programme, described earlier, was that it proved to be highly cost-effective, in addition to enhancing the participants' quality of life. The cost of the week's residential intervention per child was equivalent to only 7 hours of individual speech and language therapy in one NHS Trust. The longer the difficulties persist, the longer help is required, the more schooling is disrupted for clinical appointments and the more likely the child is to be victimised and stigmatised by peers for appearing 'different'. A vicious circle can ensue which contributes not only to the child's cycle of disadvantage, but also to continuing costs to health, education and the social services. Therefore, there is evidence of both the financial value and therapeutic value of incorporating psychosocial intervention into the clinical management of persistent communication difficulties.

Having explored some of the key psychological concepts underpinning the working philosophy, attention can be now turned to how such concepts can be put into clinical practice, which is the focus of Chapter 3.

The object of Chapter 3 is to outline the rationale and development of the activities that make up Part II of the book (the resource material). We turn our attention first to highlighting the particular advantages and disadvantages of group work, intensive therapy and residential intervention. The importance of the generalisation of learned skills and competencies following intervention is also discussed.

The rationale and development of resource material and activities

If I tell you, you will forget,

If I show you, you will remember,

If I involve you, you will understand. (anon.)

The value of group work

We spend much of our lives in social interactions of some description, both as children and as adults. For example, children mix with peers in and out of school, and with family members at home. Since these interactions are experienced in groups (of varying sizes), and since communication is the common currency by which we interact, it seems logical to manage persisting communication difficulties within a group context. As Hopson and Scally (1981, p. 112) point out:

'Whatever the task or purpose of a group, there will be a bonus of learning simply from having to act and interact with one another. . . . Perhaps if one were to identify the one skill most crucial for individuals to develop, for many it would be how to be effective in the groups in which we live, play and work.'

The authors emphasise how much can be learned from group membership that cannot easily be learned from other therapeutic contexts.

Group therapy is a highly effective means of helping communicatively-impaired young people. Small-group work, in particular, offers participants the opportunity for ample practice in fundamental communication skills, such as turn-taking (Rustin and Kuhr, 1999, p. 87). It is promising to see the emphasis being placed on co-operative work in groups, and on speaking and listening within the new National Curriculum. McCaffrey (1993, p. 132) points out that this positively encourages schools to consider how they can develop children's communication competence. Indeed, the 'Speaking and Listening' attainment target of the National Curriculum focuses on the social process, that is, the 'act of communication itself' (Fleming et al., 1997, p. 8). This, in theory, can only bode well for those with persistent communication difficulties.

O'Rourke and Worzbyt (1996, p. 5) encapsulate the essence of group work with children experiencing similar difficulties, and pinpoint that groups prove most successful when the participants:

- feel safe and secure within their group
- share a common understanding of their problem (condition)
- learn new and more effective ways to manage their situation
- express their feelings, thoughts, and diverse points of view
- experience constructive and non-judgemental feedback throughout the change process
- experience a positive self-image and personal pride
- support and encourage each other in trying new ways of thinking, feeling, and acting as they discover self-qualities and abilities previously unknown.

The group facilitator has a key role as a catalyst for nurturing personal growth in the children, by creating and sustaining the necessary environment for positive change to occur. In addition to providing a forum for obtaining new information and skills (such as sound work), groups provide a conducive psychological and physical climate for children to feel good about themselves, and all that that can empower them to do (O'Rourke and Worzbyt, 1996, p. 4).

In our experience of running residential programmes, the optimum number for whole-group sessions is 12 children, with a group leader and key helpers (some of whom need to be fully qualified). The helpers can play a significant role in observing and helping particular children during each session. Their observations enrich subsequent discussion of each child's progress amongst staff. The whole group can then be subdivided into smaller groups of 3–4 children, which appears to be the size most conducive to addressing topics in more detail, especially those of a more sensitive nature. Each of the smaller groups works concurrently on a different activity, relevant to each child's particular needs. This type of organisation also enables children to move from one group to another. Examples of whole-group and small-group activities used in the residential programmes are given later in this chapter in discussing the background on Part II activities (Table 3.3).

The many potential advantages of undertaking group work in speech and language intervention are indicated in Table 3.1. Clearly, there are also disadvantages in undertaking group work which need to be recognised: there is less individual attention for each child, and confidentiality is harder to maintain. However, in our experience, the advantages far outweigh the disadvantages.

The reader's attention is drawn to Hopson and Scally's comprehensive discussion of group work, in their seminal text on teaching lifeskills (1981, especially Chapter 5, pp. 111–203 – Working with groups in the classroom), and the excellent discussion by Rustin and Kuhr (1999, Chapter 5 – Group Therapy, pp. 56–70) on considerations for undertaking group therapy with speech-impaired children, and matters relating to group structure, planning and design.

The value of intensive therapy

There is surprisingly little reference to intensive speech and language therapy in the literature, given the unquestionable benefits of this form of intervention (outlined in Table 3.1). The possible disadvantages of intensive intervention also need to be acknowledged, such as the fact that some children may require more time between clinical sessions to consolidate newly acquired skills and competencies. The progress made during intensive intervention depends, in part, on the nature of the relationship between therapist and child. With careful and sensitive management, these issues can be addressed effectively if and when they arise.

The value of residential intervention

We have already identified the pressing need to incorporate the psychosocial aspects of communication into the clinical management of persisting communication difficulties. The study of older children with persisting communication difficulties associated with cleft palate (described in Chapter 1) has demonstrated a means by which this need can be addressed. In doing so, it aims to begin the process of reversing the victimised, ostracised and stigmatised (VOS) cycle of disadvantage, as discussed in Chapter 2.

The residential intervention study highlights the unique value of small-group work, especially within a residential context, the main advantages of which are outlined in Table 3.1. The disadvantages of residential intervention include possible homesickness, the need to detach from the group at the end of the programme and the reliance on others to maintain the progress made during the week after completion of the programme. However, in our experience, these disadvantages, which can be sensitively addressed as part of the programme, are clearly outweighed by the many advantages.

When the particular strengths of group work and residential intervention are combined,

Table 3.1 Potential advantages of group, intensive and residential forms of intervention

Potential advantages of intervention *Please note that the following examples illustrate advantages particular to one of the forms of intervention (columns). That is, not all examples are necessarily appropriate to all forms of intervention*	Form of intervention			
	Group work	Intensive therapy	Residential intervention	Non-residential intensive intervention
Psychosocial development, for example: • Provides a safe forum for discussing bullying and other sensitive issues • Opportunities to thrive in presence of peers can enhance self-perception • Enables child to build on success of previous day's achievements • Child gains confidence from being able to cope away from home	✓	✓	✓	✓
Development of peer relations, for example: • Similar difficulties within group reassure participants that they are not alone • Children befriend each other and gain confidence in building relationships • Children motivate, praise and monitor each other	✓	✓	✓	✓
Implications for schooling, for example: • Groups run during school holidays or after school avoid school absence • Group experience may enhance group activities at school (and vice-versa) and encourages opportunity to report back to schoolteacher	✓	✓	✓	✓
Timetabling and organisation of therapists' caseload, for example: • Efficient and effective way of managing children with similar difficulties • Overcomes poor/erratic attendance of clinic appointments (e.g. 1:1 therapy) • Value of running concurrent small groups as an efficient use of resources	✓	✓	✓	✓
Implications for speech and language therapists involved, for example: • Teamwork (with children, colleagues and together) is always very rewarding • Therapists gain sense of effectiveness as child moves on more rapidly • Overcomes intensity of 1:1 therapy	✓	✓	✓	✓
Implications for parents/caregivers (and family dynamics), for example: • Parents benefit from child moving on more rapidly in therapy (see above) • Opportunity to meet other parents of children in group can be supportive • Parents benefit from break and see changes when they return (residential)	✓	✓	✓	✓
Financial advantages, for example: • Cost-effective in that a number of children can be seen together • Cost-effective in that progress can be made more rapidly • Cuts down number of journeys made by parents and children for therapy	✓	✓	✓	✓

a very effective and motivating programme of therapy can emerge. In addition, the memory of having had an enjoyable, supportive and beneficial time away from home can, in itself, serve to increase the therapeutic impact of the whole experience for the children concerned.

Non-residential intensive intervention

Where residential intervention is not considered feasible or appropriate because of a child's age, the management programme being promoted can be adapted as a non-residential intensive intervention. The emphasis is still on intensive management, as this affords the opportunity for the many particular advantages of intensive group work to be experienced by the participants.

We are currently adapting the programme for use with younger children (5–7 year olds) during the early years of schooling. In view of the children's age, this would take the form of non-residential intensive intervention.

In summary, intervention can be offered to communicatively-impaired children in a variety of forms, as shown by the broad range of existing provision of speech and language therapy today. Nevertheless, speech and language therapists still make frequent use of individual one-to-one intervention. As stated above, the cost of 1 week's residential intervention per child is equivalent to only 7 hours of individual speech therapy (according to one NHS Trust). These comparisons call for further questions to be asked regarding the viability and cost-effectiveness of alternative methods of delivering speech and language therapy, especially in view of the accrued benefits of residential and intensive group contexts. The many potential advantages of undertaking non-residential intensive intervention are indicated in Table 3.1.

Generalisation of learned skills and competencies

Relatively little literature appears to be available on the matter of generalising new skills and competencies. This is surprising, as generalisation is a form of critical yardstick by which the effec-

tiveness of a particular intervention programme can be informally gauged. That is, however appropriate and sound a programme may be for a child, it cannot be considered to be effective or successful unless the progress made during the course of the intervention is maintained. This is, of course, the challenge that accompanies every form of therapy, but it is most acute in residential and intensive therapy, where claims of 'success' are linked to a short burst of intervention. This challenge is highlighted by Rustin and Kuhr (1999, p. 53) in the context of social skills training: '. . . in order for social skills training to be of worth, clients will need to demonstrate that they are able to adapt the skills taught into their everyday life in a variety of settings'.

A key feature and advantage of residential intervention is the facility to generalise what is learned in a natural setting. As soon as a session is over, the children can put into practice (and therefore reinforce), what they have just mastered by interacting with each other in 'free' periods including meal times. Such opportunities can clearly enhance the children's perception of their own capabilities, and their value should not be underestimated. Yet it is this same feature that is a primary disadvantage or shortcoming of residential work, in that its effectiveness and the maintenance of progress made is largely dependent on the extent to which the successes can be carried over into a child's daily life. Dockrell and Messer (1999, p. 150) recommend that plans for generalisation should be incorporated into the intervention programme from the start, to ensure that generalisation is feasible.

It could be argued that the degree to which achievements are generalised after attending a residential intervention programme is largely determined by the clinicians' efforts to keep in touch with the participants through, for example, evaluation questionnaires, workbooks and follow-up handouts. Such materials not only serve as reminders and motivators, but keep the experience 'alive' for the children concerned, which may be a crucial factor in maintaining progress. Where specific help is required, it is essential to share findings and recommendations with referring therapists, parents and teachers.

We were concerned by the number of children referred for the residential programme who were on review for speech and language therapy at the time. In one instance, 5 of the 12 children were reported to be on review, yet, according to our pre-intervention assessment, all of them had marked and persistent communication difficulties. This is of significance to the discussion on generalisation and maintenance of progress, since a vital part of this process is to be able to guarantee that, after attending the intervention programme, the children return to active reinforcement of newly learned skills and competencies by all involved in their welfare. In discussing therapeutic group work with children, Drost and Bayley (2001, p. 2) underline the need to put such work into perspective: 'A group is not a world in itself, it is a small moment in a child's life, a small window in a large world.' As such, it is our responsibility to make the most of that 'moment' so that its benefits can be sustained when the group has been disbanded.

It is useful at this point to consider what it is that affects the generalisation and maintenance of desirable changes and achievements made during an intensive intervention programme (both residential and non-residential). Figure 3.1 presents this process in the form of a flow chart.

If the experience of intervention is sufficiently enjoyable and memorable, it is more likely that it will make an impact on a child in terms of effecting change. If the child is then given materials and resources to keep the memory alive, it is more likely that the impact will be maintained. Therefore, we propose that it is the responsibility of parents and clinicians to keep the memory of intervention alive. There is a direct relationship between impact and maintenance. The unique features of group work and residential intervention combine to maximise the child's learning opportunity. In doing so, they also

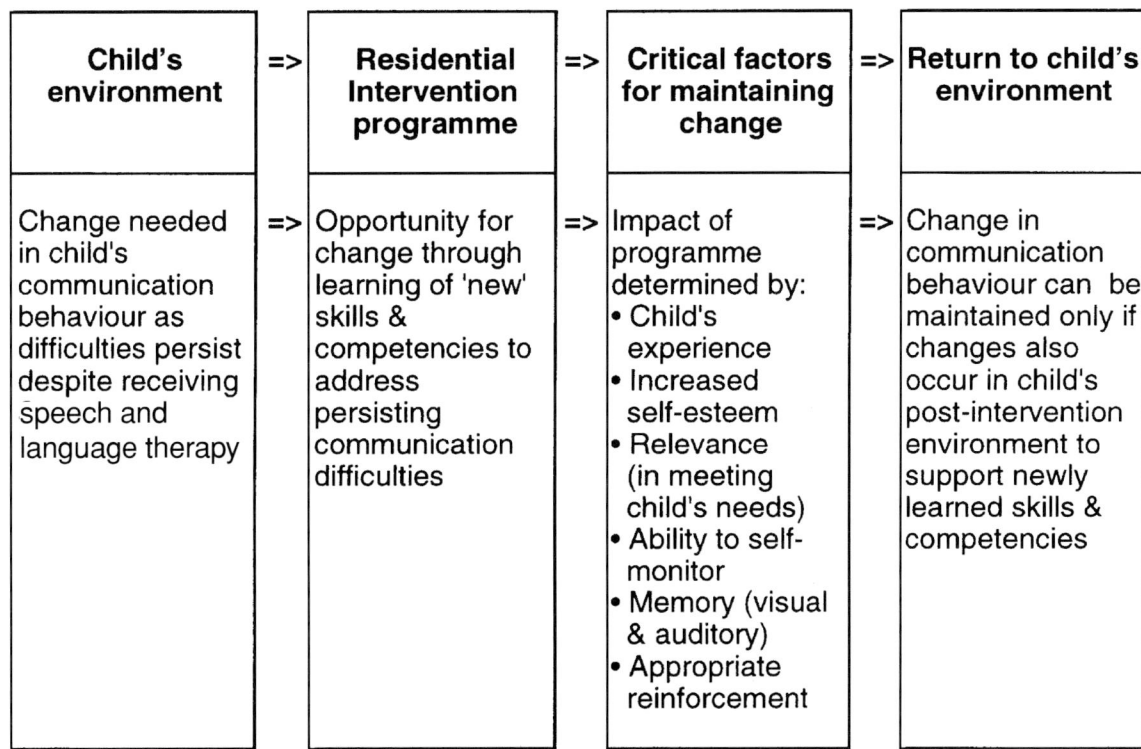

Child's environment	=>	Residential Intervention programme	=>	Critical factors for maintaining change	=>	Return to child's environment
Change needed in child's communication behaviour as difficulties persist despite receiving speech and language therapy	=>	Opportunity for change through learning of 'new' skills & competencies to address persisting communication difficulties	=>	Impact of programme determined by: • Child's experience • Increased self-esteem • Relevance (in meeting child's needs) • Ability to self-monitor • Memory (visual & auditory) • Appropriate reinforcement	=>	Change in communication behaviour can be maintained only if changes also occur in child's post-intervention environment to support newly learned skills & competencies

Figure 3.1 What determines the maintenance of progress or change?

maximise the impact of the experience for the child, because it is so meaningful and memorable.

Intensive intervention (especially residential) necessarily removes a child from their familiar environment for a period of time (i.e. longer than one-to-one half-hour regular therapy). What has changed when they return to the familiar environment? The child needs consistent support to maintain desirable changes made during the intervention, because peers and family need to be helped to acknowledge that changes have taken place, and to adapt to the child's 'new' communication behaviour (e.g. a stammerer who becomes a fluent speaker). In this sense, a further critical factor in ensuring maintenance of change is the nature of the reception the child receives from peers and family and school staff (as well as the speech and language therapist) after attending the intensive programme.

Erwin (1993) alludes to the potential difficulties of adjusting to 'new' behaviours in the context of peer relationships, and questions whether training in social skills enhances friendship or simply facilitates superficial relating. Button also considers the fundamental implications of 'progress' (1979, p. 197):

'It is not too difficult to help someone to greet, meet, and converse at a personal level with other people, but the removal of an impediment alone does not compensate for the long history of not having had practice in that give and take, equal and intimate relationship that friendship implies.'

Promoting generalisation

Rustin and Kuhr (1999, p. 54) refer to the importance of reinforcing 'new behaviours' outside therapy. In order to do this, therapists should have a sound understanding of a child's social background, and include family members, teachers and peers in considering how they can help to reinforce the child's newly acquired skills. For young children, parents or caregivers tend to be the primary social reinforcers, but the onus shifts to peers in the case of adolescents. As clinicians, we need to ask ourselves if we know enough about the child's background to promote generalisation in this way.

Erwin (1993, p. 236) also underlines the particular role played by peers in enhancing the likelihood of generalisation:

'The peer group will often function as a more natural means of delivering reinforcement and provide greater stability of outcomes (Strain and Fox, 1981). Even if the intervention is based on adults dispensing major reinforcements, ultimately peer interaction must depend on peer responses – these are the universal constituent of peer social interactions, and these are probably the crucial element in the maintenance of the benefits of an intervention.'

Alongside the support offered by family members and peers, a child's own self-monitoring and self-reinforcement are crucial factors. Meichenbaum (1986) suggests that one way of promoting long-term effects is by emphasising the part played by self-monitoring and self-reinforcement, even if the new behaviour is ignored or punished by others. In this sense, children learn to become their own therapist or teacher, which is integral to self-efficacy (as outlined in Chapter 2). In this context, Klaber Moffett and Richardson (1997, p. 89) note: '. . . self-efficacy or the patient's perception of control over the problem and ability to cope are considered important predictors of a successful outcome (for example, Johnston et al., 1992).'

In similar vein, Rustin and Kuhr (1999, p. 25) note that Bandura's (1977) analysis of self-regulatory processes (cognitive behaviour theory), stems from the notion that all changes in voluntary behaviour are mediated by the individual's perceptions of their own capability to carry out the behaviour in question (self-efficacy). Therefore, self-efficacy appears to be largely determined by self-perception, which in turn is related to self-esteem. This is evidenced by the fact that self-efficacy can be hampered by negative beliefs and unrealistic expectations. Brumfitt (1999, p. 6) also alludes to the link between self-esteem, self-perception and self-efficacy:

'. . . the individual's belief about personal effectiveness is an important aspect of the self-concept and self-esteem. If an individual feels a sense of competence for an ability that is personally valued (e.g. the ability to speak in public when the individual views that as an important ability) then this will contribute to a feeling of high self-esteem.'

Background to development of activities and resource material

In developing the material for the residential intervention programme, we paid particular attention to the process underlying the programme, in terms of the most expedient way in which to present the activities to the children. This was crucial if each child was to gain the optimum benefit from attending the programme. Since the participants were not only of different ages, but also had different capabilities, the programme was designed to start with material that was relevant to all the children, whatever their age or communication difficulties. By starting from general and progressing to more individualised and specific activities, we felt that the group had a common base point to refer to, as necessary, during the course of the week.

The purpose of this section is to offer some guidance on implementing each of the sections in Part II, and to pinpoint the significance of each of them to the management approach being promoted. Reference is first made to how the residential programme fitted together to incorporate both psychosocial and speech production aspects of communication.

For the residential intervention programme, the four experienced speech and language therapists (all members of the research team), took responsibility for planning and leading activities for different identified needs, although all were involved in every aspect of intervention, whether it was related to communication or psychosocial adjustment. This was essential because here we had the unique opportunity to live with the children for a short time, and in that time to help them to open the door to change.

In planning the programme, we prepared a summary of each participant including two aims; one focusing on perceived psychosocial needs and one on communication. We also specified objectives. This exercise led to the development of a matrix of needs for the whole group, which also identified the needs of each child (Table 3.2). From this matrix, it is evident that all of the children needed to relax, to speak out, to use repair strategies, to improve their oral awareness and to improve listening skills.

Indeed, this is probably true for all children with communication difficulties. Ten of the children needed articulation help, with four trying out the use of electropalatography (EPG). All but two children presented with marked psychosocial needs. The matrix of needs provided an important planning tool for the activities for the week. The profiles of two children on the programme are outlined below.

Profile of Child A

This child was 14 years old, with a history of bilateral cleft lip and palate. At referral Child A was receiving regular speech and language therapy, and had done so intermittently since infancy. There were considerable difficulties regarding articulatory/phonetic patterns, with persistent use of double articulation involving the glottis. Child A tried hard to produce 'correct' sounds but created excess tension and then involved the glottis in doing so. Phonetic realisations varied. There was a need to move the focus of articulation away from the glottis, to the front of the vocal tract. The introduction of EPG was considered the best way to try to change a deeply entrenched and inappropriate pattern. There was also evidence of hyper-nasality and some audible nasal emission.

Child A had a complex and turbulent home background, and also reported persistent bullying by peers both inside and outside school. In adopting a retaliatory way of coping with these experiences, this child was becoming disruptive and getting into trouble with school staff. Maintaining friendships was also problematic.

Aims and objectives for Child A (following pre-intervention assessment)

Communication:

- to help Child A use best communication skills in a relaxed manner
- to reduce tension in speech by looking at relaxation techniques
- to look at gentle production of bilabial placement, i.e. silent mouthing
- to use EPG to look particularly at alveolar placement
- to look at and employ repair strategies

Psychosocial:

- to enable Child A to become a more confident communicator
- to equip Child A with effective coping strategies for handling bullying.

Profile of Child B

Child B was a 13-year-old adolescent with a history of unilateral cleft lip and palate and severe speech difficulties. At referral, Child B was on review regarding speech and language therapy, and had received therapy intermittently since infancy. Articulation involved persistent palatal/velar/glottal placements and variable phonetic realisations. There was also evidence of double articulation, severe hypernasality, audible nasal emission and nasal grimace. Child B's poor intelligibility was exacerbated by speaking too quickly and with marked tension. With a short and very scarred soft palate, the adequacy of velopharyngeal closure was questionable. There was a marked class III occlusion. During assessment, there was a notable discrepancy between Child B's performance on the simple sentence repetition task and spontaneous speech.

Child B's home background was unsettled and complex. In 'coping' with the diverse communication and psychosocial difficulties, it appeared that Child B had learned some maladaptive survival strategies. This gave the child the appearance of being 'streetwise' and able to cope with anything. Further observation showed that Child B clearly lacked self-confidence and had a fragile self-esteem with poor social skills. This child also spoke of being bullied by peers.

Aims and objectives for Child B (following pre-intervention assessment)

Communication:

- to enable Child B to use appropriate speech and communication skills more consistently
- to work on bilabial and labiodental placement to try to reduce double articulation
- to look at tongue tip contact for /t/ and /d/

- to work on 'speaking out' strategies e.g. slowing down, mouth opening, volume
- to look at and employ repair strategies
- to reduce tension in speech by working on relaxation techniques

Psychosocial:

- to enable Child B to become a more confident communicator
- to equip Child B with effective coping strategies for handling bullying.

The residential intervention programme

The residential programme took place in the school summer holiday, and ran from Sunday afternoon to the following Friday late afternoon. On day 1 of the course the children were brought by their parents or caregiver, who were invited to spend approximately 3 hours with us. The speech and language therapist assigned as the key person to take particular 'intervention' responsibility for a child, discussed aims and objectives with the child and their parents or caregiver (Table 3.2). Each therapist had special responsibility for three children. The parents were seen as a group and given an overview of the week's programme, while the children got to know each other and the student helper assigned to take special care of them in intervention as well as in social activities. The student also carried out the appropriate follow-up activities with the child concerned.

During the week, much of the time was spent in whole-group sessions, where many of the children's identified needs could be addressed collectively. The days generally followed the same pattern, starting and ending with a whole-group relaxation session, followed by the day's various activities. A time for reflecting on each child's achievements was also built into the end of each day. During this time each child was encouraged to say what they had been most proud of achieving that day. This whole-group session became known as 'Prouding time'. This particular activity proved to be one of the most significant ways of raising the participants' levels of

Table 3.2 Matrix of individual needs – residential intervention programme, July 1999

Child	SO	R	RS	OA	EPG	A	LA	LI	SS	SC	SEC	MFO	GA	TB
1	✓	✓	✓	✓	×	✓	✓	✓	✓	✓	✓	✓	✓	✓
2	✓	✓	✓	✓	×	✓	×	✓	✓	✓	✓	✓	✓	✓
3	✓	✓	✓	✓	×	✓	×	✓	✓	✓	✓	✓	✓	✓
4	✓	✓	✓	✓	✓	×	×	✓	✓	×	×	×	×	×
5	✓	✓	✓	✓	✓	✓	×	✓	✓	✓	✓	✓	✓	✓
6	✓	✓	✓	✓	×	×	✓	✓	✓	✓	✓	✓	✓	✓
7	✓	✓	✓	✓	✓	✓	✓	✓	✓	✓	✓	✓	✓	✓
8	✓	✓	✓	✓	✓	✓	×	✓	✓	✓	✓	✓	✓	✓
9	✓	✓	✓	✓	×	✓	✓	✓	✓	✓	✓	✓	✓	✓
10	✓	✓	✓	✓	×	✓	×	✓	✓	✓	✓	✓	✓	✓
11	✓	✓	✓	✓	×	✓	✓	✓	✓	✓	✓	✓	✓	✓
12	✓	✓	✓	✓	×	✓	×	✓	×	×	×	×	×	×
Total	12	12	12	12	4	10	5	12	11	10	10	10	10	10

✓ = identified need; × = not an identified need.
SO, speaking out; R, relaxation; RS, repair strategies (what to do if the other person cannot understand you); OA, oral awareness; EPG, electropalatography (a computer-based resource for working on articulation of specific sounds); A, articulation (without EPG); LA, language; LI, listening; SS, social skills (eye contact and turn-taking); SC, self-consciousness; SEC, self-esteem and self-confidence; MFO, making friends and relating to others; GA, group activities; TB, teasing or bullying

self-esteem and self-perception, in addition to self-monitoring and self-evaluation.

Notes on the progress of each child were updated on a daily basis by members of the research team, and the four student helpers were encouraged to record their observations in the appropriate files. The period after the children had gone to bed provided a valuable opportunity to discuss their progress, and to amend the programme for the following day if necessary. By participating with the children in daily activities, such as mealtimes, outings, shopping and picnics, everyone was involved in the social fabric of the residential experience. In doing so, clinicians and helpers accrued a sense of what it must be like to live with a persisting communication difficulty on a daily basis. We also caught a glimpse of what it is to live with a communicatively-impaired child. Table 3.3 shows how the different activities on the residential programme were organised.

How aims and objectives were addressed in the residential programme

The large, open, flexible space in the purpose-built school unit allowed us to work with different groups of children concurrently, as well as enabling the children to move around the appropriate groups. There was also sufficient space for individual sessions to discuss feelings and anxieties. The availability of space is, therefore, a key factor in being able to run concurrent sessions. Table 3.4 shows the programme for the residential week.

Objective-focused activities were interspersed with free times, treat times and lots of food and drinks. At post-intervention assessment, every child said that they had enjoyed the week, an essential ingredient in enabling the development of confidence and self-esteem and triggering change. All team members saw as central the necessity of building warm, supportive and trusting relationships with the children.

On the last day of the course, the Emotional Behaviour Scales used for pre-intervention assessment were repeated. The children again watched a video cartoon and retold the story individually. The communication data were audio and video recorded (as outlined in Chapter 1).

Parents arrived after lunch and joined us for around 3 hours for debriefing. Each child and parent was seen by their key member of staff, and the progress and recommendations discussed. The research team met with the whole group of parents to share activities carried out in the week,

Table 3.3 Organisation of different activities on the residential programme

Whole group activities	Small group activities	Individual 1 : 1 activities

Relaxation
Coping with teasing/bullying
'Prouding' (positive self-image)
Talking about feelings
Oral awareness
Repair strategies
Social skills
Speaking out and voice hygiene
	Articulatory/phonetic aspects
	Articulation – using EPG
	Coping with teasing/bullying
	Talking about feelings
	Phonology
	Language
	Listening
	Speaking out and voice hygiene
	Whisper techniques
	Soft vocal attack
	Intonation (all supra-segmental
	    elements)
	Transfer of new patterns
	    into daily speech
		Electropalatography (EPG)
		Coping with teasing/bullying
		Talking about feelings

Table 3.4 Programme for the residential intervention week

Time	Monday	Tuesday	Wednesday	Thursday	Friday
9.00	The mouth and making puppets	What did we learn yesterday and what are we going to do today?	Whole group relaxation and voice loudness range	Relaxation and voice	8.30 – Relaxation and Prouding time
9.30		Relaxation	Small groups	Bullying and teasing	Bullying – whole group
10.00–10.10		Talking about feelings			Watch video
10.30			Drinks		
11.00	Having fun with smiling	Small groups – individual progress	Small groups continue	Communication – small groups	Individuals
11.30					
12 noon	Free time	Free time		Free time	
12.30	Lunch	Lunch	Picnic lunch		Lunch
1.00					
1.30	Start diaries	Small groups continue	Interviews in pairs	Communication – small groups	Pack and tidy up
2.00–2.15	Swindon Football Club	Whole group meets			Parents arrive
2.30	Drinks and diaries	Drinks and diaries	Drinks	Drinks	Feedback to parents/caregivers
3.00	Drinks	Drama	Art	Drama	
3.30	Speaking out				Tea
4.00–4.15	Did your message get across?				
4.30	Tea (cooked meal)	Walk to shops	Drinks and cakes and start diaries	Interviews continued	Goodbye
5.00		(postcards, ice creams)			
5.30	Music band	Tea (cooked meal)	Pond dipping and fishing	Diaries, Prouding and tidy up	
6.00				Visitors arrive for barbecue	
6.30	Free time	Free time	Fish and chip shop		
7.00	Free time	Being proud			
7.30	What have we done well today ('Prouding time') and diaries	Write postcards, Prouding time and diaries	Free time, Prouding time and diaries		
8.00					
8.30	Drinks and biscuits		Drinks and biscuits		
9.00			Relaxation		
9.30	Goodnight!		Goodnight!		

and to encourage continued and appropriate support of the children. This was particularly important in relation to vocal abuse and coping with bullying. A 'Communication Activities Book' was developed out of the programme and was sent to the children shortly after they returned home. The activities book was the key to the development of the resource material in Part II.

After the course, a full report was prepared for each child and sent to the referring speech and language therapists. The main areas recommended as ways forward are outlined below.

'Opening the door' to effective communication: recommended ways forward

The unique value of small-group work in a supportive environment is recommended for carrying out the intervention procedures outlined below.

- Recommended approaches for increasing volume, directing airflow through mouth and reducing hypernasality and glottali-sation:
  - relaxed speaking out with wide mouth opening
  - soft vocal attack
  - speaking out with appropriate speed and good intonation
- Whisper speech technique to encourage precise articulatory contact, and reduce abuse of the vocal tract and larynx
- Continuing with Electropalatography where indicated (EPG)
- Communication repair strategies
- Recommended approaches for building-up a child's self-esteem, and perception of self as someone with whom it is worth communicating:
  - development of self-monitoring skills
  - focus on personal strengths
  - social skills (eye contact, listening, etc.)
  - use of strategies for coping with bullying and enhancing social competence.

The following section shows examples of the recommendations made for Child A and Child B, whose profiles and aims and objectives for the residential programme were outlined earlier.

Recommendations made for Child A

From observations and intensive work with Child A during the residential programme, the team recommended various ways forward. These included the continued use of a relaxed approach to speaking, with soft vocal attack, and whispering technique, which proved beneficial in establishing consistent and appropriate phonetic realisations and excluding double articulation. The further use of EPG was also strongly recommended in view of the benefits accrued during the residential week.

With respect to psychosocial functioning, by the end of the programme Child A felt that effective coping strategies for handling bullying had been learned. It was recommended that these be put into practice with the start of the new school term. There was little doubt that Child A became a more confident communicator in the course of the week, particularly regarding achievements made with EPG and speaking out in group sessions about experiences of being bullied. This child's increased self-confidence and self-perception was apparent to all. The importance of continued work in both these areas was highlighted by the team.

Recommendations made for Child B

From observations and intensive work with Child B during the residential programme, the team recommended the use of relaxation, soft attack, speaking out and whispering techniques. Intensive periods of intervention during school holidays were advised in view of the diversity of Child B's communication and behavioural difficulties (which became increasingly more apparent as the residential week progressed).

During the week, Child B became a more competent communicator in speaking out and in generalising work achieved in increasing speech intelligibility. This was particularly evident after relaxation exercises. It was suggested that progress in these areas be continued, to maintain improved self-confidence and self-esteem. It was also considered desirable for this child to internalise work done on coping with bullying, in order to put the coping strategies into action when required.

In conclusion

In these first three chapters, we have sought to outline the working philosophy of a team of experienced speech and language therapists, who feel like Edward Bear in the introduction to Chapter 2, that 'there really is another way' (A.A. Milne, Winnie the Pooh). On this occasion, the opportunity to undertake a continuing research project has enabled us to 'stop . . . and think' of how persistent communication difficulties might best be managed in school-aged children in mainstream education.

Having discussed the working philosophy in the light of various sources of literature, and described the rationale and development of the activities which reflect the philosophy, it is now time to introduce the activities that comprise the resource material of Part II. We very much hope that these activities will prove to be enjoyable, beneficial and illuminating to all involved.

4　Introduction to resource material

In this introduction to the resource material, we highlight the pertinence of each section to our recommended management approach. The activities comprising the resource material are based on our clinical and educational experience, with particular reference to the 1996 and 1999 residential programmes for children with persisting communication difficulties (as outlined in Chapter 1).

Organisation of the resource material

The resource material is organised in eight sections which are listed below, and subsequently discussed in further detail. The sequence of the sections reflects the underlying process of the intervention programme. That is, high priority is given first to creating a safe and supportive environment for the children, before embarking on areas which are both sensitive and very personal to the children (such as experiences of being bullied at school).

It should be noted that the sections and related activities have been devised in such a way that the sheets can be used either in their chronological order, or as stand-alone activities according to a child's particular needs. The sheets can be photocopied as required for use in group work, and for individual follow-up.

We would like to emphasise that the programme is intended for use with children and adolescents aged 7–16 years, in mainstream education. This is ambitious, in view of the developmental changes that take place within this age range. Nevertheless, great care has been taken to offer maximum flexibility and scope within the programme, since youngsters can differ widely in their communicative competence and psychosocial functioning, which may not be representative of their chronological age. The activities in each section follow a logical sequence. The nature of the material in some of the worksheets means that they make more complex conceptual demands on the child. The adult working with the child will know where it is necessary to provide further explanations, and ensure that the child understands what to do before the sheet is given as a follow-up activity.

Although the activities in each section follow a logical sequence, they are not designed to increase in difficulty. Indeed, we have deliberately not been prescriptive in indicating age levels for the activities, since the clinicians implementing the programme will be sensitive to each child's needs and capabilities. Having said this, the successful accomplishment of any of the activities can help to enhance a child's self-perception and belief that they can do it.

Content of the resource material

The activities comprising the resource material reflect our underlying working philosophy: that persistent communication difficulties can be most expediently addressed by incorporating the wider psychosocial aspects of communication into a child's clinical management. That is, if psychosocial functioning is optimised alongside attention to speech (and other features of communication), the child will be motivated by an enhanced sense of personal worth and purpose. By addressing these fundamental needs, real progress in communication competence can be made, since communication is essentially about our ability to relate to others and enjoy rewarding friendships.

Embedded in the suggested activities are the notions that:

- each child is different
- each child may be at a different stage
- it is alright for a child not to be able to do something
- being different is special
- self-evaluation is essential to progress
- activities can be fun.

The sections of the resource material are as follows:

Introductory sheet for those helping child at home or at school
Section 1   Ice-breaking and discussing group 'ground rules'
Section 2   Using relaxation to keep calm
Section 3   Feeling good about yourself
Section 4   Getting out of difficulties (e.g. teasing and bullying)
Section 5   How your voice works
Section 6   Sending messages through speaking
Section 7   What to do if your message is not understood
Section 8   Making the best use of your voice and speech

As the participants may not have met before joining the programme, the initial ice-breaking activities serve to introduce the children and participating adults to each other, in a gentle and non-threatening way (section 1). The establishing of 'ground rules' for the group by the children, enables the group to develop an identity of its own, where the participants can be at ease with each other, and where, at a later stage, personal difficulties can be expressed with minimum awkwardness.

Introducing simple relaxation exercises early on in the programme gives the children the opportunity to 'unwind' and to reduce any fears and anxieties about their communication difficulties. Having focused on reducing tension and then promoting a positive self-image, it is then feasible to look at effective coping strategies for handling difficult situations, such as being bullied (sections 2–4, psychosocial aspects). The

remaining four sections (5–8) centre on communication, and show the sequence in which different features, including speech production, are introduced to the participants. As noted before, in the context of intensive intervention, the two aspects of the intervention (psychosocial and communication) can be concurrently addressed in the programme.

With respect to the assessment and evaluation of a child's progress on the programme, the importance of encouraging self-monitoring skills is apparent throughout the sections. In some instances, this takes the form of evaluation activities or a quiz within the group. In others, the daily recording of reinforcement activities at home or school is recommended. We are undertaking the development of a formal battery of scales for assessing progress as part of our ongoing research study.

By way of preparing to implement the programme, it may be useful for the clinicians involved to consider the following issues for each of the children concerned:

- How do they perceive their own abilities to speak or communicate?
- How do they cope on a daily basis with persisting communication difficulties?
- How are they getting on at school?
- Do they have a circle of good friends at school and at home?
- Are they bullied about their speech or the way they communicate with others?
- How do they self-monitor or evaluate their own progress?
- What is their home situation?

Section 1
Ice-breaking and discussing group 'ground rules'

Rationale
The purpose of the initial ice-breaking activities is to introduce everyone in an informal and enjoyable way, so that everyone feels at ease within the group. Once introductions have been completed, the group can have fun deciding what their ground rules should be. The setting of ground rules from the start conveys messages to

the children regarding the value of respecting others, and behaving and communicating in a socially acceptable way.

Outline of activities

Adherence to the agreed rules is likely to be much higher if the children have thought of them themselves. However, the following ideas could be encouraged:

- Each person is a valuable member of the group.
- Be kind to one another.
- Only one person should speak at a time (so no interrupting).
- Everything said in the group is confidential (and therefore private within the group).

Section 2
Using relaxation to keep calm

Rationale

A child who is fearful and anxious about anything will not fully benefit from any help being offered. Therefore, it is the clinician's responsibility to maximise the learning opportunity, by creating as conducive and worry-free an environment as possible. The child may not only be distracted by being away from home, but on a more chronic level, may be harbouring the build-up of bodily tension associated with having a persisting communication difficulty. Unless this tension is addressed, it will gradually accumulate and continue to hamper the child's progress. It may also bring other stress-related symptoms in its wake, such as headaches, sickness and a range of ailments.

The purpose of this section is to increase awareness of the body and how it reacts to difficult situations, so that the children can gain control over these reactions. More precisely, equipping children with relaxation skills encourages them to recognise bodily cues related to stress and anxiety, and promotes a tangible means of combating such feelings. In this way, fundamental lifeskills can be learned at an early age, and the children can become increasingly competent in dealing with difficult situations.

Outline of activities

There are now many resources available for those wishing to know more about relaxation, but these resources are generally targeted at adults rather than children. And yet, if we could encourage children to master simple relaxation techniques, this would not be so alien to them as adults. The key to enabling children to do this effectively is to keep the techniques simple and memorable. Further information on the stress cycle and the 'fight or flight' mechanism which underpins all relaxation techniques, can be found in the Further Reading section.

In introducing Sheet 2.2 to the participants (derived from Atherton, Calm Kids Cope, p. 25), clinicians may like to explain the reasons for what happens to the body when we feel worried and tight inside. Table 4.1 shows part of the body's fight-or-flight response to stress (derived from Nash, 2000).

Table 4.1 What happens to the body when we feel worried and tight inside

Effect on body	Why this happens
Hair stands on end	To speed heat loss
Mouth feels dry	Appetite repressed
Shoulders are raised	Tension to prepare the body for action
Breathing is faster	More oxygen for energy
Heart beats faster	Blood circulates oxygen quicker to muscles
Hands are sweaty	Perspiration increased to cool body in action
Tummy feels tight	Digestion restricted as energy directed to muscles
Legs feel tight	Tension to prepare the body for action

In order to benefit from relaxation sessions, the children need to understand the concept of relaxation at the outset. Care should be taken in the choice of words used to convey the sensations of stress versus relaxation (constriction and release of tension respectively)

The simple relaxation procedure used on the residential programme (sheets 2.3a and 2.3b) proved to be an effective way of helping the participants to distinguish between the tightness associated with stress and tension, and the calm, comfortable feeling of being relaxed. Once children have mastered even the basics of relaxation techniques, they can be encouraged to use them on a regular basis as part of speech and language therapy and at home and school, especially when encountering threatening and difficult situations (such as bullying).

A quiet, dimly lit environment is most conducive to relaxation. Ideally, the instructor's voice should be slightly monotonous, slow and calm. The use of gentle, calming music can be a helpful aid.

Section 3
Feeling good about yourself

Rationale

The importance of raising a child's self-esteem and self-perception for enhancing communication competence has been already discussed in Chapter 2. In this section of the resource material, suggestions are made as to how this theory can be put into practice. Part of this process involves helping the youngsters to develop their sense of self, by identifying their own characteristics and personal preferences (such as in choosing hobbies), and by being aware of their particular strengths and weaknesses.

Outline of activities

A range of different activities is recommended for promoting a positive self-image. Initially, the focus is placed on the participants thinking about themselves (Sheets 3.1–3.3 and 3.7). Examples of these include identifying characteristics and good points about oneself. Other activities incorporate the writing of a daily journal to record personal

achievements and progress during the programme and 'Prouding time' sessions, in which the children are encouraged to say what they have been pleased about doing.

Next, attention is turned to how we relate to others and how we make and keep friends, since it is largely friends with whom we choose to communicate (Sheets 3.4–3.6b). In this way, fundamental lifeskills can be developed in undertaking these activities. The use of video recording is also recommended to enable the participants to monitor themselves (and others). Where the activities are derived from existing material, details can be found in Further Reading. Sheet 3.2 ('My good points' activity) is derived from O'Rourke and Worzbyt (1996, p. 362): Sheets 3.3, 3.4 and 3.6a are derived from Borba and Borba (1982, pp. 45, 19 and 43 respectively).

In the brainstorming activity suggested on Sheet 3.5, the following keys to friendship could be incorporated into the discussion.

* Talk to them and share jokes with them.
* Be kind and say nice things about them.
* Invite them to do things with you – you probably like to do the same things.
* Treat your friends how you would like to be treated yourself.
* Call them by their name.
* Show you are interested in what they say by:
  – listening to them
  – looking at them when they talk to you
  – taking turns when talking with them
  – smiling at them.

Section 4
Getting out of difficulties (e.g. teasing and bullying)

Rationale

Section 4 focuses on helping children to develop strategies for coping with difficult situations, especially teasing and bullying. By equipping children with adaptive and effective coping strategies, we can empower and enable them to become confident of their abilities to handle challenging situations as and when they arise.

Perceiving that one can cope in such situations can be a significant boost to a sense of self-efficacy and social competence.

The terms 'teasing' and 'bullying' are both used in this section, since in our experience they are often used interchangeably by the children themselves.

Outline of activities

The activities in section 4 first look at feelings associated with difficult and uncomfortable situations. By enabling the group to identify and acknowledge these feelings, it is possible to address the more sensitive issues surrounding teasing and bullying in subsequent sheets.

Sheet 4.6 shows an adapted version of the force-field technique of visualisation as used on the residential programme (see Further Reading). On these occasions, after an introductory discussion, the children were invited to make paper darts and to write on them all the hurtful names that they had been called. A member of staff then put on a black dustbin bag to represent the individual who had been bullied. It was suggested that if the darts were hurled at the person, they would not penetrate the dustbin bag and therefore not injure the person inside. In this way, the hurtful comments on the darts were seen to bounce off the vulnerable person and fall on the ground (no more than 'puffs of air'). A further whole-group discussion followed these activities, and it was emphasised that this way of coping with bullying needed practice in order to think about the hurtful comments in this way. This proved to be a useful activity in demonstrating how the children could take charge of difficult situations, by learning how to respond (adaptive), rather than react (maladaptive), to these challenging situations. It is notable that it became one of the most vividly recalled activities in the follow-up evaluations of the programme.

The section ends with suggestions about how to memorise what to do in difficult circumstances. If the activity is sufficiently memorable, there is more chance that the group members will be able to 'learn' what to do and then to put it into practice when necessary.

Section 5.
How your voice works

Rationale

The purpose of section 5 is to help the participants to develop a thorough understanding of how their voice works, as a prerequisite for sound-based therapy. In doing so, a picture can be built up of how the voice relates to speech, and why it is so important to care for the voice.

Outline of activities

A number of children with speech difficulties at the articulatory and phonetic level also have dysphonia. This is because these youngsters tend to try extra hard to make themselves understood and use excess effort, which can affect their whole body, to produce clear speech (as found in children with VPI, hearing loss or cerebral palsy). Excess effort, together with overuse of the glottis as an articulator, is vocally abusive and is likely to lead to dysphonia.

If dysphonia develops, a vicious circle can ensue, because a child who does not obtain the desirable sensory feedback may use excess effort in producing voice, thus leading to unnecessary forcing and tension. The consequent compensatory and maladaptive habits can be hard to break. Dysphonia adds to the communication deficit and may be a long-term risk. For further information see Stengelhofen (1990, 1993). Therefore, although the worksheets are devoted to voice, it must be remembered that the voice cannot be separated from the articulatory and resonatory levels.

Section 6
Sending messages through speaking

Rationale

Section 6 is concerned with sound-making. The activities in this section are based on the concept that if children are to move forward in improving specific speech skills, it is essential that they are equipped with a clear understanding of the way speech works.

Outline of activities

The suggested activities should enable children to explore where and how sounds are made. The difference between long and short consonants is emphasised, although phonetic terms such as plosive and fricative are not used. Voiced and voiceless pairs are also given considerable attention. Where neurological or anatomical factors contribute to a child's speech and communication deficits, the signalling of the difference between voiced and voiceless pairs may present major difficulties. In some children (for instance those with cerebral palsy, cleft palate or velopharyngeal incompetence [VPI]), the whole of the vocal tract may be functioning inappropriately and abusively, leading to added speech difficulties. Examples of this are where the glottis may be used as a frequent place of articulation to achieve plosion, or where the tension involved in trying to communicate may lead to vocally abusive behaviour in general, with consequent dysphonia.

The children are encouraged to carry out the suggested activities with a helper, who could be an adult (parent, teacher or speech and language therapist). However, children in groups can and often do help each other, and they can be matched for complementary skills. Where activities are complex, the supervising adult should check that the task is fully understood before children continue on their own. Where listening activities are suggested, the clinician will be in a position to decide when a child should move on to sound production (after liaison with parents and teachers).

Identifying where and how speech sounds are made

The activities in section 6 include questions that encourage children to think about and evaluate their own abilities and progress. We also hope that the material will stimulate different ways of thinking about the role of speech in communication. For example, with respect to oral awareness, what level of knowledge and understanding can and should we presume a child to have? If erroneous assumptions have been made about their depth of knowledge, it is conceivable that they may have received months or even years of speech and language therapy, without fully grasping what is required and why they need therapy in the first place.

If children can be encouraged early on to become active partners rather than receptive clients, a joint exploration of where sounds are made will help them gain both knowledge and understanding from the outset. One means of doing this is to immerse them in a sensory experience of sound where all the senses can be seen to be working together, before starting to work directly on sounds. In implementing the suggested activities, children will gain a thorough understanding of where and how speech sounds are made by being able to visualise, hear and feel properties of those sounds (for example, by looking into each other's mouths and exploring what different sounds 'look' like). The experience of sound is made real by demystifying the mouth, and explaining and demonstrating what speech sounds are all about. Moreover, once the children fully understand the process by which sounds are made, they are in a position to internalise that understanding and experience every time they open their mouth to work on sounds (Figure 4.1).

If the foundations of speech skills are laid down in this way, children can develop a much clearer idea of the purpose of therapy and what they are required to do by the speech and language therapist. As a result, they are motivated and can become competent and confident learners in the process. The implications of this approach for enhancing a child's self-perception as someone who can achieve should not be underestimated.

An example of how this framework can be put into practice is in the use of electropalatography (EPG), which was used with great enthusiasm and success on the residential programme. It proved particularly beneficial in helping the older children with persisting communication difficulties to break through a

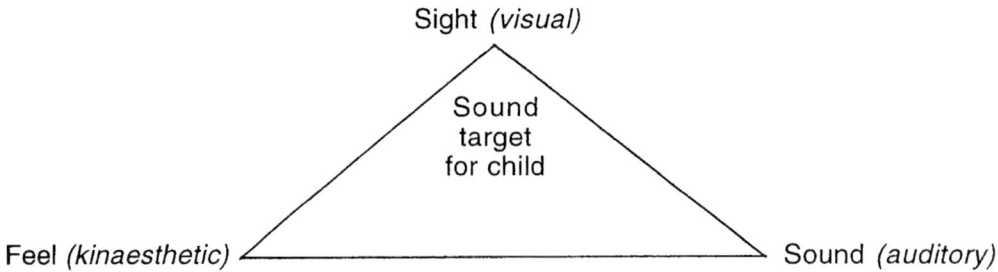

Figure 4.1 Child's sensory experience of sound.

plateau in their progress. EPG is motivating for the participant in several ways:

- novelty value (computer-based therapy)
- multi-sensory feedback (auditory, visual and kinaesthetic)
- enables children to self-monitor and evaluate their own progress
- helps children understand what is going on inside their mouth
- encourages children to persist and try to improve on previous performance (like many computer-based games).

More information on the use of EPG can be found in Further Reading.

The sound chart (Sheet 6.4b), based on the International Phonetic Alphabet, is designed primarily for English speakers (although it will allow for the addition of some non-English sounds). It focuses on the place of articulation, because introducing manner of articulation would make the chart too complicated for phonetically naive children and for most parents and caregivers.

As earlier activities in section 6 encourage children to explore sounds used by other speakers (such as classmates), it is important for children from other language backgrounds to be able to gain greater insight into their own sound-making, and to plot their own phonetic inventory. The use of correct symbols is not important, but marking the chart for the place of articulation, and being guided by an informed adult about manner, could be of immense value. For this reason, a blank chart

which incorporates both place and manner of articulation is included, and provides the opportunity to plot sounds from any language (Sheet 6.4c, derived from the International Phonetic Alphabet), for example:

- the place retroflex is important with / ʈ ɖ ɳ ɽ / all using this position (e.g. Urdu, Punjabi)
- the lateral fricative /ɬ/ used rarely in English is found in Welsh
- the linking of the plosives /t/ with /d/ and /k/ with /g/ in Arabic
- the two types of roll in Czech, where alveolar roll /r/ contrasts with post-alveolar roll /ɾ̠/

It is advisable to spend time with parents and carers identifying the sounds expected in a child's first language, so that non-English sounds can be recognised as appropriate for that language, and not attributed to a phonetic or articulatory difficulty. The recognition of difficulties of production across different languages (for example, the absence of fricatives), can provide greater insight into the exact nature of a child's difficulties at articulatory, phonetic and phonological levels.

The borrowing of sounds from one language to another needs to be acknowledged and accepted as a very usual process. How many adult and fluent speakers do we know who still have strong accents and persisting use of sounds from another language, but are nevertheless effective communicators?

Section 7
What to do if your message is not understood

Rationale

When children find that other people cannot understand what they are saying, the experience can be deeply frustrating and bewildering for the individuals concerned (for both speaker and listener). Therefore, an essential part of the 'tool kit' for those with persistent communication difficulties is to know what to do if and when such experiences arise. The main purpose of this section is to provide children with a variety of communication 'tools', which together will enhance overall confidence and competence in communication and lead to more intelligible speech.

Outline of activities

This section focuses on the options available, and offers various strategies which the group can enjoy learning and putting into practice. The suggested activities may be especially useful as a means of enthusing demotivated youngsters who may despair at their inability to make themselves understood by others. Some individuals give up the struggle more easily than others, and even fool themselves into thinking that communicating with other people does not matter that much.

In considering other ways of getting our message across, the suggested activities encourage the group to think about the options in helping other people to understand them better. The significance of social skills, such as listening and body language, are highlighted as particularly valuable repair strategies.

The features shown in Figure 4.2 can all play a part in improving speech intelligibility. By raising the profile of these dimensions, the pressure is taken off 'speech' per se and children can gain confidence in their own competence as communicators. For example, if children 'can do' activities for varying volume of sound, their confidence is boosted by knowing that they have just grasped a fundamental dimension of speech.

Section 8
Making the best use of your voice and speech

Rationale

Part of communicating effectively and confidently is the knowledge that we are communicating as

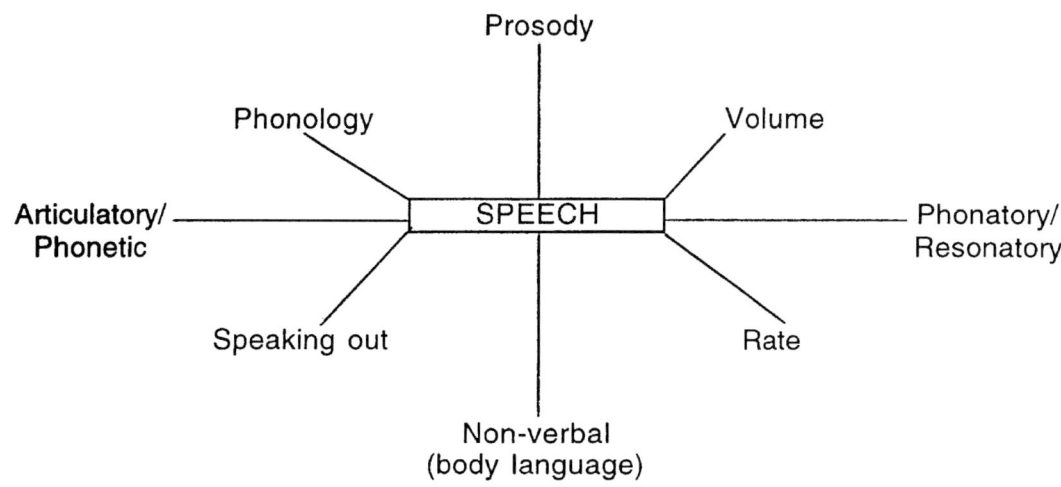

Figure 4.2 Features contributing to intelligibility of speech.

well as we can. The rationale behind Section 8 is the belief that children can be encouraged to think about the range of communication skills they have at their disposal, and to recognise where and when they are not using them to the best of their ability. By maximising the skills they have, individuals should find that they have a greater chance of being understood by others and, thereby, of experiencing rewarding communication with others.

Outline of activities

In helping children to make the best use of their voice and speech, it is crucial to remember that each child's own individual strengths must be taken into account. What may help one child may not be what helps another. Facilitating 'best' speech is therefore very much about individualising the repertoire of skills in accordance with each child's needs and competencies. For example, where a child is trying so hard to be understood that dysphonia develops (see Section 5), the most pertinent advice may to encourage the child to stop trying to talk so clearly. This may be the key to a more relaxed approach to communicating, thereby unblocking some significant obstacle.

With respect to the suggested activities, the skills needed for optimising 'best' speech which are advocated in the activities include:

- looking up
- opening mouth
- using the best articulation the child can manage
- using eye contact

- using appropriate volume
- using appropriate rate
- using appropriate intonation patterns.

In undertaking the activities, a first priority is to raise the children's confidence and competence as effective communicators. A greater understanding of the mechanisms of speech production, and the communicative context in which speech is used, can enhance the feeling of being in control and the perception of being an effective communicator. Moreover, intelligibility of speech may be improved in the process and even as a result of focusing on other aspects of communication for a while. Indeed, working on speech alone is unlikely by itself to bring about a functional change in a persistent communication problem. This is borne out by the fact that the difficulty may persist at school age despite hours and even years of therapy. Within this framework, we need to adopt a 'bottom-up' paradigm (Figure 4.3).

And finally …

This resource material was developed by the combined efforts of the research team, in devising a programme for children with persisting communication difficulties as part of a research study. This study is ongoing, and as the potential scope of the programme for different client groups becomes increasingly apparent, the resource material will be continually appraised and expanded. We would welcome any comments or observations from those implementing the material, and would be happy to discuss any aspect of the programme in further detail.

Increased likelihood of a competent communicator who is now enabled to tackle challenging aspects of speech and language therapy

Start by building up child's strengths, knowledge, confidence and understanding in the process of communication

Figure 4.3 Giving priority to psychosocial aspects of communication.

Further reading and resources

Many texts and materials have proved valuable in preparing this publication and devising the residential intervention programme. A collection of them are cited here for those wishing to pursue further reading.

Useful references and resources

Bullying and handling difficult situations

The references given below offer further insight into the background and management of bullying. Bradbury gives a concise description of the force-field technique, and illustrates how it can be implemented with children. Cooper's article contains some very helpful ideas on developing resilience in coping with difficult situations. Cowie, Katz et al. and Luthar et al. also contribute to the literature on how to manage bullying effectively. The article by Mooney and Smith has direct relevance for speech and language therapists in understanding the impact of bullying upon those with dysfunctional communication. Sharp offers insights into her clinical work on counselling bullied students and provides a valuable framework for such intervention.

There are various titles available for children which focus on bullying; a collection of these can usually be found in the children's section of local libraries (or under information for parents). Examples of these are the books by Bottner and Grunsell noted below.

Bottner B (1992) Bootsie Barker Bites. Mammoth, London.

Bradbury E (1996) Counselling People with Disfigurement. British Psychological Society Books, Leicester.

Cooper C (2000) Discovering resilience to disfigurement. The New Therapist 7(3): 31–33.

Cowie H (2000) Bullying: the challenge of peer support. The New Therapist 7(4): 30–33.

Grunsell A (1995) 'Let's Talk About' – Bullying. Gloucester Press, London.

Katz A, Buchanan A, Bream V (2001) Bullying In Britain, Testimonies from Teenagers. Report produced by Young Voice and The Centre for Research Into Parenting and Children, Department of Social Policy and Social Work, Oxford University. Young Voice, Surrey.

Luthar SS, Cicchetti D, Becker B (2000) The construct of resilience: a critical evaluation and guidelines for future work. Child Development 71(3): 543–562.

Mooney S, Smith PK (1995) Bullying and the child who stammers. British Journal of Special Education 22(1): 24–27.

Sharp S (1998) Chris, Usha and Bridget: supporting bullied students. In: Syder D (ed) Wanting To Talk, Counselling Case Studies In Communication Disorders. Whurr, London.

Cleft palate

The following books focus on the management of cleft palate. Nash looks at the psychosocial implications, and highlights the everyday experiences of those born with a cleft. Stengelhofen offers a clear and comprehensive guide for those working with cleft-impaired patients (1990). The texts by Stengelhofen (1993) and Watson et al. (2001) examine the wider implications of cleft palate and the importance of adopting a multi-disciplinary approach to management.

Nash P (1995) Living With Disfigurement: Psychosocial Implications of Being Born With A Cleft. Avebury, Aldershot.

Stengelhofen J (1990) Working With Cleft Palate. Winslow Press, Bicester.

Stengelhofen J (1993) The nature and causes of communication problems in cleft palate. In: Stengelhofen J (ed) Cleft Palate: The Nature and Remediation of Communication Problems. Whurr, London

Watson A, Sell D, Grunwell P (2001) Management of Cleft Lip and Palate. Whurr, London.

Communication difficulties and social skills

The following references offer a variety of resource material. McCroskey and Beatty's journal article reports on research findings, whereas the texts by House and Morris and Rustin and Kuhr offer practical ideas for working with children within a theoretical framework. Dockrell and Messer outline different language and communication problems and discuss key elements of intervention. Fleming et al. focus on speech and language difficulties in the context of the child's education, and the interface between speech and language therapy and school.

Dockrell J, Messer D (1999) Children's Language and Communication Difficulties, Understanding, Identification and Intervention. Cassell, London.

Fleming P, Miller C, Wright J (1997) Speech and Language Difficulties in Education. Winslow Press, Bicester.

House H, Morris J (1997) Let's Communicate, A Handbook for People Working With Children With Communication Difficulties. World Health Organization, Geneva.

McCroskey JC, Beatty MJ (1984) Communication apprehension and accumulated communication state anxiety experiences: a research note. Communication Monographs 51: 79–84.

Rustin L, Kuhr A (1999) Social Skills and the Speech Impaired (2nd ed). Whurr, London.

Electropalatography (EPG)

Hardcastle et al. provide a useful introduction to EPG, and Gibbon and Crampin document a specific application of EPG with a cleft-impaired patient.

Gibbon F, Crampin L (2000) An instrumental investigation of mid dorsum palatal stops in an adult with repaired cleft palate. Paper presented at the Annual Conference of the Craniofacial Society of Great Britain and Ireland, Reading.

Hardcastle W, Morgan Barry R, Nunn M (1993) Instrumental articulatory phonetics in assessment and remediation: case studies with the electropalatograph. In: Stengelhofen J (ed) Cleft Palate the Nature and Remediation of Communication Problems. Whurr, London.

Group work with children

These resources offer a wealth of material for group work with children within a theoretical framework. Drost and Bayley present their activities according to two age bands (5–7 and 8–11 year olds). In each case, they advocate a 10-session intervention programme. The material is aimed at building up the social, interpersonal and emotional skills of children with behavioural difficulties, but it has direct relevance for those working with communicatively-impaired children. O'Rourke and Worzbyt organise their material according to particular areas of need, such as social skills and stress management. In each instance, the practical activities are preceded by background information and a discussion of the rationale, with guidelines for implementing the material. Both texts are very useful resources for group work with children and the activities can be adapted where necessary.

Drost J, Bayley S (2001) Therapeutic Groupwork with Children. Speechmark, Bicester.

O'Rourke K, Worzbyt JC (1996) Support Groups for Children. Accelerated Development, London.

Relationships with peers

Erwin's book offers valuable insights into the development and nature of peer relationships. It also discusses how and why problems can arise in children's relationships, and how they can be managed.

Erwin P (1993) Friendship and Peer Relations in Children. Wiley, Chichester.

Relaxation with children

There appear to be very few resources which directly address relaxation methods for children. The materials listed below offer comprehensive and straightforward techniques which can be used with school-aged children in groups.

Atherton M (no date given) Calm Kids Cope. Helping Children with Stress. Calm Kids Company Limited and Stress Management Training Institute (Registered Charity No. 264906).

Nash W (1998) At Ease with Stress, the Approach of Wholeness. London: Darton Longman and Todd.

Self-esteem and self-concept

The majority of references below are practical resource materials, which offer innovative ways to enhance the self-esteem and self-concept of children (Borba and Borba, Canfield and Wells and Hartley-Brewer). Brumfitt and Hopson and Scally address the psychosocial development and functioning of children from different perspectives. Brumfitt highlights the importance of raising self-esteem and self-concept in managing communication difficulties. Hopson and Scally, on the other hand, focus upon the relevance of these life skills to the child's education and general development. The Changing Faces publication is one of a series of booklets designed for the facially disfigured, which has direct relevance for all those working with children with low self-esteem and a poor self-perception (see section on useful contacts below to purchase booklets).

Borba M, Borba C (1982) Self-Esteem: A Classroom Affair. More Ways to Help Children Like Themselves. Harper and Row, San Francisco.

Brumfitt S (1999) The Social Psychology of Communication Impairment. Whurr, London.

Canfield J, Wells HC (1976) 100 Ways To Enhance Self-Concept In the Classroom, A Handbook for Teachers and Parents. Prentice-Hall, Englewood Cliffs, NJ.

Changing Faces publication (1998) Looking Different Feeling Good! (see contact details below).

Hartley-Brewer E (2000) Self Esteem for Boys, 100 Tips for Raising Happy and Confident Children. Vermilion, London.

Hartley-Brewer E (2000) Self Esteem for Girls, 100 Tips for Raising Happy and Confident Children. Vermilion, London.

Hopson B, Scally M (1981) Lifeskills Teaching. McGraw-Hill, London.

Voice

The treatment of voice disorders in children and adolescents is always a challenge for the speech and language clinician. The book by Andrews and Summers provides a clear account of normal voice changes and the conditions which affect vocal behaviour in adolescents. Evaluation is covered comprehensively and includes useful case examples. The sections on intervention are particularly valuable and include detailed examples of practice materials. It is a very good clinical resource book.

Andrews M, Summers A (1988) Voice Therapy for Adolescents. College-Hill Publication, Boston, MA.

Useful addresses and contact details

Cleft Lip and Palate Association (CLAPA)
Registered charity founded by members of staff at Great Ormond Street Hospital, London.
235–237 Finchley Road,
London, NW3 6LS.
Tel: 020 7431 0033
Website: www.clapa.cwc.net
Email: clapa@cwcom.net

Amongst other literature, CLAPA produces a magazine called Left Clip twice a year; this is primarily written for and by children and adolescents with a cleft (email: leftclip@clapa.com).

Changing Faces
Registered charity founded by James Partridge in 1992 for the facially disfigured. Information, social skills workshops, counselling and advice.
1 & 2 Junction Mews,
London, W2 1PN.
Tel: 020 7706 4232
Website: www.changingfaces.co.uk
Email: info@changingfaces.co.uk

Let's Face It
Registered charity founded by Christine Piff in 1983 for the facially disfigured. Information, counselling support network.
14 Fallowfield, Yateley,
Hampshire, GU46 6LW.
Tel: 01252 879630
Website: www.letsfaceit.force9.co.uk
Email: betsyletsfaceit@post.com

Kidscape
Registered charity founded by Michelle Elliott in 1984. Information and guidance on child safety and bullying (e.g. anti-bullying programmes for schools)
152 Buckingham Palace Road,
London, SW1W 0DH.
Tel: 020 7730 3300
Website: www.kidscape.org.uk
Email: contact@kidscape.org.uk

Royal College of Speech and Language Therapists
2 White Hart Yard,
London, SE1 1NX.
Tel: 020 7378 1200
Website: http:/www.rcslt.org.uk
Email: postmaster@rcslt.org

Young Voice
Registered charity. Listening and responding to young people.
12 Bridge Gardens,
East Molesey,
Surrey, KT8 9HU.
Tel: 020 8979 4991
Website: www.young-voice.org

References

Albery EH (1986) Type and assessment of speech problems. In: Albery EH, Hathorn IS, Pigott RW (eds) Cleft Lip and Palate: A Team Approach. Wright, Bristol.

Albery L, Chapman R (1979) Intensive speech therapy for children. In: Ellis RE, Flack FC (eds) Diagnosis and Treatment of Palato-Glossal Malfunction. College of Speech Therapists, London.

Asher SR, Coie JD (eds) (1990) Peer Rejection in Childhood. Cambridge University Press: Cambridge.

Atherton M (no date given) Calm Kids Cope. Helping Children with Stress. Calm Kids Company Ltd and Stress Management Training Institute. Registered Charity No 264906, Freephone (UK) 0800 3891800.

Bandura A (1977) Self-efficacy: Toward a unifying theory of behavioral change. Psychological Review 84: 191–215.

Bandura A (1986) Social Foundations of Thought and Action: A Social Cognitive Theory. Prentice Hall, Englewood Cliffs, NJ.

Bandura A (1997) Self-Efficacy: The Exercise of Control. WH Freeman, New York.

Bandura A, Taylor CB, Williams SL, Mefford IN, Barchas JD (1985) Catecholamine secretion as a function of perceived coping self-efficacy. Journal of Consulting and Clinical Psychology 53: 406–414.

Beitchman JH, Hood J, Inglis A (1990) Psychiatric risk in children with speech and language disorders. Journal of Abnormal Child Psychology 18: 283–296.

Bishop DVM (1997) Uncommon Understanding Development Disorders of Language Comprehension in Children. Psychology Press, Hove.

Blatchford P (1992) Academic self assessment at 7 and 11 years: Its accuracy and association with ethnic group and sex. British Journal of Educational Psychology 62: 35–44.

Borba M, Borba C (1982) Self-Esteem: A Classroom Affair. More Ways to Help Children Like Themselves. Harper & Row, San Francisco.

Bronfenbrenner W (1979) The Ecology of Human Development. Harvard University Press, Cambridge, MA.

Brumfitt S (1999) The Social Psychology of Communication Impairment. Whurr, London.

Brumfitt SM, Sheeran P (1999) VASES: The Visual Analogue Self-Esteem Scale. Winslow Press, Bicester.

Button L (1979) Friendship patterns. Journal of Adolescence 2: 187–199.

Cairns RB, Cairns BD (1988) The sociogenesis of self concepts. In: Bolger N, Caspi G, Downey G, Moorehouse M (eds) Persons in Context. Developmental Processes. Cambridge University Press, Cambridge,.

Chesebro JW, McCroskey JC, Atwater DF, et al. (1992) Communication apprehension and self-perceived communication competence of at-risk students. Communication Education 41: 345–360.

Clarbour J, Roger D (1999) The role of social anxiety, malevolent aggression and social self-esteem in adolescent emotional behaviour. Paper presented at the British Psychological Society Developmental Section Annual Conference, September 1999, Nottingham.

Damon W, Hart D (1988) Self-Understanding in Childhood and Adolescence. Cambridge University Press, Cambridge.

Davis H, Fallowfield L (1991) Preface. In: Davis H, Fallowfield L (eds) Counselling and Communication in Health Care. Wiley, Chichester.

Department for Education and Skills (2001) Promoting Children's Mental Health within Early Years and School Settings. DfEE 0121/2001. Department for Education and Skills.

Dockrell J, Messer D (1999) Children's Language and Communication Difficulties. Understanding, Identification and Intervention. Cassell, London.

Dodge KA, Pettit GS, McClaskey CL, Brown MM (1986) Social competence in children. Monographs of the Society for Research in Child Development 51(2), No. 13.

Drost J, Bayley S (2001) Therapeutic Groupwork With Children. Speechmark, Bicester.

Durand VM, Barlow D (1997) Abnormal Psychology: An Introduction. Brooks/Cole, Pacific Grove, CA.

Durkin K (1995) Developmental Social Psychology from Infancy to Old Age. Blackwells, Oxford.

Dweck C (1999) Self-Theories: Their Role in Motivation Personality and Development. Essays in Social Psychology. Psychology Press, Hove.

Eiser C (1993) Growing Up with a Chronic Disease. The Impact on Children and their Families. Jessica Kingsley Publishers, London.

Elkind D (1988) The Hurried Child: Growing Up Too Fast Too Soon (revised ed). Addison-Wesley, Reading, MA.

Enderby P, Philipp R (1986) Speech and language handicap: towards knowing the size of the problem. British Journal of Disorders of Communication 21: 151.

Engel GL (1980) The clinical application of the biopsychosocial model. American Journal of Psychiatry 137: 535–544.

Erikson EH (1963) Childhood and Society (2nd ed). WW Norton, New York.

Erwin P (1993) Friendship and Peer Relations in Children. Wiley, Chichester.

Festinger L (1954) A theory of social comparison processes. Human Relations 7: 117-140.

Fleming P, Miller C, Wright J (1997) Speech and Language Difficulties in Education. Winslow Press, Bicester.

Frey D, Carlock CJ (1989) Enhancing Self-Esteem (2nd ed). Accelerated Development, Muncie, In.

Frydenberg E (1997) Adolescent Coping Theoretical and Research Perspectives. Routledge, London.

Gerrard JM (1991) The teasing complex in facially deformed children. Australian and New Zealand Journal of Family Therapy 12(3): 147–154.

Goodyer IM (2000) Language difficulties and psychopathology. In: Bishop DV, Leonard LB (eds) Speech and Language Impairments in Children: Causes, Characteristics, Intervention and Outcome. Psychology Press, Hove.

Harding A, Harland K, Razzell R (1996) Cleft Audit Protocol for Speech (CAPS). (Available from Speech and Language Therapy Department, Broomfield Hospital, Chelmsford, Essex, UK).

Harter S (1983) Developmental perspectives on the self-system. In: Hetherington EM (ed) Handbook of Child Psychology Vol 4 Socialization, Personality, and Social Development. Wiley, New York.

Harter S (1987) The determinants and mediational role of global self-worth in children. In: Eisenberg N (ed) Contemporary Topics in Developmental Psychology. Wiley, New York.

Harter S (1988) Developmental processes in the construction of the self. In: Yawkey TD, Johnson JE (eds) Integrative Processes and Socialization: Early to Middle Childhood. Erlbaum, Hillsdale, NJ.

Harter S (1997) The personal self in social context: Barriers to authenticity. In: Ashmore RD, Jussim L (eds) Self and Identity: Fundamental Issues. Oxford University Press, New York.

Harter S (1999) The Construction of the Self, A Developmental Perspective. Guilford Press, London.

Hartley-Brewer E (2001) Learning To Trust and Trusting To Learn: How Schools Can Affect Children's Mental Health. A paper written for the Institute for Public Policy Research.

Hattie J (1992) Self Concept. Erlbaum, Hove.

Heatherton T, Ambady N (1993) Self-esteem, self-prediction, and living up to commitments. In: Baumeister R (ed) Self-Esteem: The Puzzle of Low Self-Regard. Plenum Press, New York, pp. 87–111.

Hill EL (2001) Non-specific nature of specific language impairment: a review of the literature with regard to concomitant motor impairments. International Journal of Language and Communication Disorders 36(2): 149–171.

Holland S (2000) Promoting Mental Health. Community Practitioners and Health Visitors' Association, London.

Hopson B, Scally M (1981) Lifeskills Teaching. McGraw-Hill, London.

Horne MD (1985) Attitudes Towards Handicapped Students: Professional, Peer and Parent Reactions. Erlbaum, Hillsdale, NJ.

Huskie CF (1979) Intensive therapy - Glasgow experience. In: Ellis RE, Flack FC (eds) Diagnosis and Treatment of Palato-Glossal Malfunction. College of Speech Therapists, London.

Hymel S, Franke S (1985) Children's peer relations: assessing self-perceptions. In: Schneider BH, Rubin KH, Ledingham JE (eds) Children's Peer Relations: Issues in Assessment and Intervention. Springer, New York.

Johnston M, Gilbert P, Partridge C, Collins J (1992) Changing perceived control in patients' with physical disabilities, an intervention study with patients receiving rehabilitation. British Journal of Psychology 32: 89–94.

Kaplan H, Martin S, Johnson R (1986) Self-rejection and the explanation of deviance: specification of the structure among latent constructs. American Journal of Sociology 92: 384–441.

Kapp-Simon KA, McGuire DE (1997) Observed social interaction patterns in adolescents with and without craniofacial conditions. Cleft Palate-Craniofacial Journal 34: 380–384.

Kapp-Simon K, Simon D, Kristovich S (1992) Self-perception social skills adjustment and inhibition in young adolescents with craniofacial anomalies. Cleft Palate-Craniofacial Journal 29: 352–356.

Kish V, Garlick W (1999) Managing the psycho-social aspects of visible difference: an evaluation of self-help booklets for young people. Paper presented at the 6th European Craniofacial Congress, 1999, Manchester UK.

Klaber-Moffett JA, Richardson PH (1997) The influence of the physiotherapist-patient relationship on physical disability. Journal of Physiotherapy Theory and Practice 13: 89–96.

Kobasa S (1979) Stressful life events, personality, and health: an inquiry into hardiness. Journal of Personality and Social Psychology 37: 1–11.

Lewis M (1990) Social knowledge and social development. Merrill-Palmer Quarterly 36: 93–116.

Lindsay G, Dockrell J (2000) The behaviour and self-esteem of children with specific speech and language difficulties. British Journal of Educational Psychology 70: 583–601.

Lipowski ZJ (1986) Psychosomatic medicine: past and present. Part I. Historical background. Canadian Journal of Psychiatry 31: 2–7.

Liptak GS (1987) Spina bifida. In: Hoekelman S, Blatman SB, Friedman SB, Nelson NM, Seidel HM (eds) Primary Paediatric Care. CV Mosby, St Louis.

Luthar SS, Cicchetti D, Becker B (2000) The construct of resilience: a critical evaluation and guidelines for future work. Child Development 71(3): 543–562.

Marsh HW (1985) Age and sex effects in multiple dimensions of preadolescent self-concept: a replication and extension. Australian Journal of Psychology 37: 197–204.

Marsh HW, Craven RG, Debus R (1991) Self-concepts of young children 5 to 8 years of age: measurement and multidimensional structure. Journal of Educational Psychology 83: 377–392.

McCaffrey P (1993) Groupwork with stressed children. In: Alsop P, McCaffrey P (eds) How to Cope with Childhood Stress: A Practical Guide For Teachers. Longman, Harlow, UK.

McClelland DC (1985) The social mandate of health psychology. American Behavioral Science 28: 451–467.

McCroskey JC, Beatty MJ (1984) Communication apprehension and accumulated communication state anxiety experiences: a research note. Communication Monographs 51: 79–84.

Meichenbaum D (1975) Enhancing creativity by modifying what subjects say to themselves. American Educational Research Journal 12: 129–45.

Meichenbaum D (1986) Cognitive behaviour modification. In: Kanfer FH, Goldstein AP (eds) Helping People Change: A Textbook of Methods (3rd ed). Pergamon Press, New York.

Mooney S, Smith PK (1995) Bullying and the child who stammers. British Journal of Special Education 22(1): 24–27.

Mruk C (1999) Self-Esteem Research Theory and Practice (2nd ed). Free Association Books, London.

Nash P (1995) Living with Disfigurement: Psychosocial Implications of Being Born with A Cleft Lip and Palate. Avebury, Aldershot.

Nash P, Kellow B, Toombs L, Brown J, Stengelhofen J (1997) Preliminary report on evaluating the effect of a residential holiday programme for the total communication needs of children with cleft palate. Paper presented at the Annual Conference of the Craniofacial Society of Great Britain , 1997, Chelmsford UK.

Nash P, Stengelhofen J, Toombs L, Brown J, Kellow B (2001b) An alternative management of older children with persisting communication problems. Proceedings of the Royal College of Speech and Language Therapists Conference, 2001, Birmingham UK. International Journal of Language and Communication Disorders. Supplement 36, 179-184.

Nash P, Stengelhofen J, Toombs L, Brown J, Kellow B (2001c) National survey of children aged 8-18 years with persisting communication problems associated with cleft palate. Child Language Teaching and Therapy 17(1): 19–34.

Nash W (1998) At Ease with Stress, the Approach of Wholeness. Darton Longman and Todd, London.

Nash W (2000) Stress management training programme. Unpublished.

O'Rourke K, Worzbyt JC (1996) Support Groups for Children. Accelerated Development, London.

Parker JG, Asher SR (1987) Peer relations and later personal adjustment: are low-accepted children at risk? Psychological Bulletin 102: 357-389.

Pelham BW, Swann WB (1989) From self conceptions to self worth: on the sources and structure of low self esteem. Journal of Personality and Social Psychology 57: 672-680.

Putallaz M, Gottman J (1981) Social skills and group acceptance. In: Asher S, Gottman J (eds) The Development of Children's Friendships. Cambridge University Press, Cambridge.

Rice ML, Sell MA, Hadley PA (1991) Social interactions of speech and language impaired children. Journal of Speech and Hearing Research 34: 1299–1307.

Roger D (1992) The development and evaluation of a work skills and stress management training programme. Paper presented at the Annual Conference of the British Psychological Society, 1992, Scarborough.

Roger D (1997) Managing Stress: The Challenge of Change. Chartered Institute of Marketing, Maidenhead.

Rosenberg GM (1979) Conceiving the Self. Basic Books, New York.

Rosenberg M (1986) Self-concept from middle childhood through adolescence. In: Suls J, Greenwald AG (eds) Psychological Perspective on the Self (Vol. 3). Erlbaum, Hillsdale NJ.

Roskies E, Lazarus RS (1980) Coping theory and the teaching of coping skills. In: Davidson P, Davidson S (eds) Behavioral Medicine: Changing Health and Lifestyles. Bruner/Mazel, New York.

Rubin KH, Stewart SL (1996) Social withdrawal. In: Mash EJ, Barkley RA (eds) Child Psychopathology. Guilford Press, London.

Ruble DN (1994) A phase model of transitions: cognitive and motivational consequences. Advances in Experimental Social Psychology 26: 163–214.

Ruble DN, Thompson EP (1992) The implications of research on social development for mental health: an internal socialization perspective. In: Ruble DN, Costanzo PR, Oliveri ME (eds) The Social Psychology of Mental Health: Basic Mechanisms and Applications. Guilford, New York.

Rustin L, Kuhr A (1999) Social Skills and the Speech Impaired (2nd ed). Whurr, London.

Rutter M (1985) Resilience in the face of adversity. Protective factors and resistance to psychiatric disorder. British Journal of Psychiatry 147: 598–611.

Rutter M, Rutter M (1992) Developing Minds, Challenge and Continuity Across the Life Span. Penguin, London.

Sarafino EP (1990) Health Psychology: Biopsychosocial Interactions. Wiley, New York.

Schultz NR, Moore D (1989) Further reflections on loneliness research. In: Hojat M, Crandall R (eds) Loneliness: Theory Research and Applications. Sage, Newbury Park, CA.

Schwartz GE (1982) Testing the biopsychosocial model: The ultimate challenge facing behavioral medicine? Journal of Consulting and Clinical Psychology 50: 1040–1053.

Seiffge-Krenke I (1990) Developmental processes in self-concept and coping behaviour. In: Bosma H, Jackson S (eds) Coping and Self-Concept in Adolescence. Springer, New York.

Seligman ME (1975) Helplessness. WH Freeman, Reading, MA.

Seligman M (1995) The Optimistic Child. Random House, NSW Australia.

Sell D, Harding A, Grunwell P (1999) GOS.SP.ASS.'98: an assessment for speech disorders associated with cleft palate and/or velopharyngeal dysfunction (revised). International Journal of Language and Communication Disorders 34: 17–33.

Sheridan CL, Radmacher SA (1992) Health Psychology, Challenging the Biomedical Model. Wiley, Chichester.

Smith PK (1999) England and Wales. In: Smith PK, Morita Y, Junger-Tas J, Olweus D, Catalano R, Slee P (eds) The Nature of School Bullying, A Cross-National Perspective. Routledge, London.

Snowling MJ, Adams JW, Bishop DVM, Stothard SE (1999) Educational attainment of school leavers with a preschool history of speech-language impairments. International Journal of Language and Communication Disorders 36(2): 173–183.

Stackhouse J, Wells B (1998) Psycholinguistic Assessment of Children with Speech and Literacy Difficulties. Whurr, London.

Stengelhofen J (1990) Working with Cleft Palate. Winslow, Bicester.

Stengelhofen J (ed) (1993) Cleft Palate: The Nature and Remediation of Communication Problems (2nd ed). Whurr, London.

Strain PS, Fox JJ (1981) Peers as behavior change agents for withdrawn classmates. In: Lahey BB, Kazdin EE (eds) Advances in Clinical Child Psychology Vol 4. Plenum Press, New York.

Sylva K (1994) School influences on children's development. Journal of Child Psychology and Psychiatry 1: 135–170.

Taylor SE, Brown JD (1988) Illusion and well-being: A social psychological perspective on mental health. Psychological Bulletin 103: 193–210.

Tennen H, Affleck G (1993) The puzzles of self-esteem: A clinical perspective. In: Baumeister R (ed) Self-Esteem: The Puzzle of Low Self-Regard. Plenum Press, New York.

Thomas PT, Turner SR, Rumsey N, Dowell T, Sandy JR (1997) Satisfaction with facial appearance among subjects affected by a cleft. Cleft Palate-Craniofacial Journal 34: 226–231.

WHO (1980) International Classification of Impairments, Disabilities and Handicaps. World Health Organization, Geneva.

resource
material

Improving Children's Communication
Managing Persistent Communication Difficulties

Pop... & Louise Toombs

WHURR PUBLISHERS
London & Philadelphia

Improving communication
Information for parents/carers/teachers

NAME: DATE:

As we know, speaking and communicating is harder for some people than others; both young people and adults.

Some have particular difficulties that persist in spite of a lot of effort from the people themselves and those around them. The cause of the problems may be obvious, or it may be unknown.

These young people may have worked for many years to improve the way they speak. They may have felt isolated and had difficulty making friends. They may have been teased or bullied. Their poor self-image can hamper further progress.

The aim of this programme is to help young people make the best of what they have, in order to communicate more easily, in other words to help them develop some empowering strategies to break out of this vicious cycle.

Each section focuses on an area of need, for example, relaxation, specific speech sounds, enhancing self-esteem and dealing with bullying.

As the adults around them, you can help by taking an interest in what they are doing, and being aware of the strategies they are learning. It is hard work for them, but it is easier if they know that others are helping them to take responsibility for their own communication.

Schoolteachers
It may be that you could use some of the ideas for discussion in groups, as all of us would benefit from better communication skills, and this may help to reduce the isolation felt by a young person.

(Child's name) .... is learning about:

How you can help
Please ask the speech and language therapist if you have any questions about this, or if you would like to know more about the programme.

Your comments:

section 1

Ice-breaking and discussing group 'ground rules'

1.1 Hello, who are you?

When we meet new people, it is a good idea to introduce ourselves and to tell them a little bit about us, such as our name and what we enjoy doing (our hobbies and interests). They may then tell us their name and say a bit about themselves. In this way, we can begin to make friends with them. Introductions are an important way of getting to know the others in your group. Have some fun trying the following activities and introducing yourselves to each other.

NAME: DATE:

ACTIVITY For this activity, you will need a bean bag or something soft that you can throw to each other. Sit in a circle (at the table or on the floor), one person volunteers to start this activity by saying 'Hello I'm (your name), who are you?' and then throws the bean bag to someone in the group (preferably somebody the person does not already know). The person who catches the bag then does the same, 'Hello I'm (your name), who are you?' and so on until everyone knows each other's name. The activity gets faster as the bag-throwing speeds up.

ACTIVITY **What do you enjoy doing most?**

On a sheet of paper, jot down three things that you really enjoy doing.

When you have done this, fix your sheet of paper to the board, so that all the sheets can be seen easily and everyone in the group can read them. Write your initials beside each activity that you enjoy doing too. Have a go and see who enjoys doing the same things as you in your group.

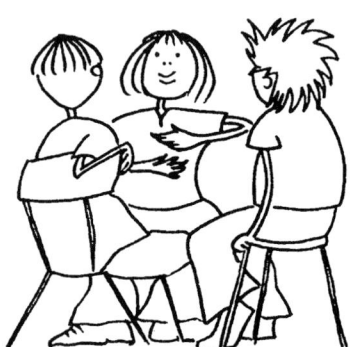

My name is ...., do we share the same interests?

	I really enjoy	We really enjoy doing that too (initials of others in group)
1.		
2.		
3.		

1.2 Why we need 'ground rules' for the group

Now that you know who else is in the group, think about what sort of rules you would like to have for the group. It is important for any group of people to agree on certain rules and to try hard to keep them, so that the group can work well together and enjoy doing the same activities.

NAME: DATE:

ACTIVITY   **What rules are important for this group?**
A good way to start talking about rules for the group is for everyone to stop and think for a moment, and then to say what they have thought about. This is called brainstorming and can be great fun. Everyone can have a go and tell the rest of the group what rules they think are important. For example, is it important to be nice and kind to everyone in the group? If so, say so!

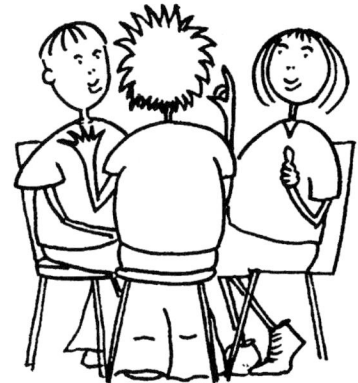

The rules for this group
1.
2.
3.
4.
5.
6.
7.
8.
9.
10.

section 2

Using relaxation to keep calm

2.1 Why we need to relax and keep calm

Do you know what the word relaxation means? It means calming down so we feel less tight inside, and not so worried about things. It is an important word to remember, because:

- Relaxation helps us to calm down when we have feelings we don't like, such as feeling worried and scared if we are teased or bullied by others.
- Did you know that when we are worried and scared, our bodies get tight and feel all knotted up inside?
- Once we know about what happens to us, we can learn to do some simple exercises, which can really help us to feel better and happier inside.

NAME: DATE:

ACTIVITY   **What happens to us when we are worried and tight inside?**
Its useful to know about this, so let's spend a bit of time working it out. Write down your ideas in the boxes below. When you have finished we can talk about them in the group, and see if other people have written down the same things as you.

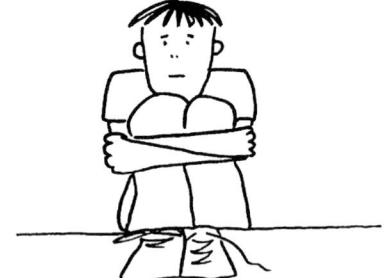

> How do you feel when you are worried and tight inside?
> (For example, do you feel cross and bad tempered, and feel like crying?)
>
> *
> *
> *

> What happens to your thinking when you are worried and tight inside?
> (For example, can you think clearly or remember things well?)
>
> *
> *
> *

> How do you behave towards others when you are worried and tight inside?
> (For example, do you want to be alone and not talk to other people?)
>
> *
> *
> *

2.2 What happens to our bodies when we feel worried and tight inside?

You may like to put this poster up in your bedroom to remind you that whenever you feel worried and tight inside you say to yourself:

I need to RELAX!

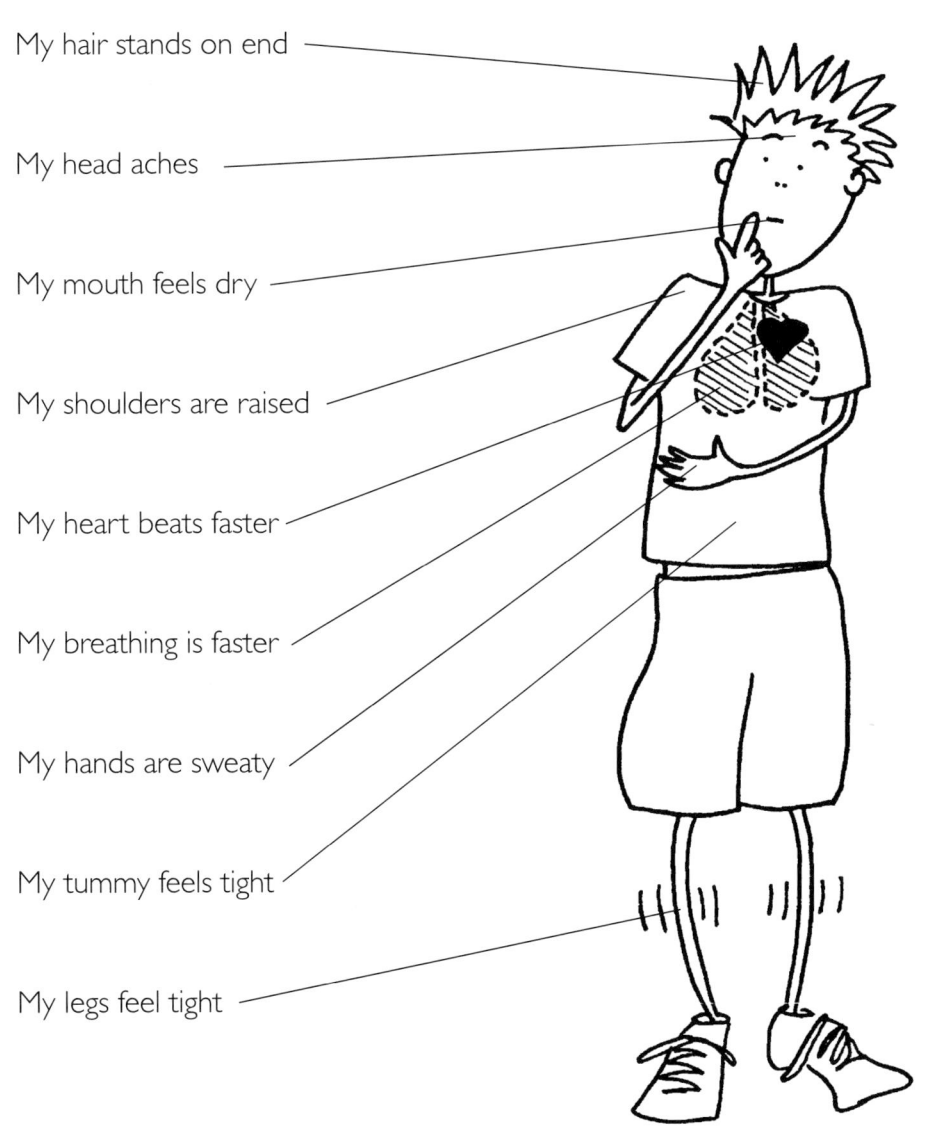

My hair stands on end

My head aches

My mouth feels dry

My shoulders are raised

My heart beats faster

My breathing is faster

My hands are sweaty

My tummy feels tight

My legs feel tight

2.3a Twelve steps to help us to keep calm

NAME: DATE:

ACTIVITY   This is a useful activity to do first thing in the morning and before you go to bed, and when you are trying to use your best talking skills. It will help you to feel the difference between tightness in your hands and shoulders, and the lovely feeling of relaxing as you let go of the tightness. You may like to ask someone else to do it with you.

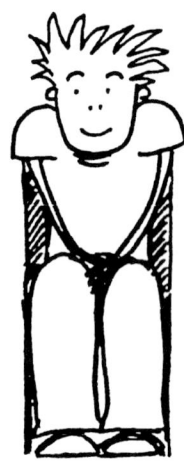

You may feel all tight inside at the start of this activity

Step 1   To do this relaxation exercise sit comfortably in a chair. Can you remember the words 'bottom back' as a way of getting into a good position on the chair? Put your feet flat on the floor and your hands on your lap.

Step 2   To calm your body down, sit quietly and count backwards from 10 (10, 9, 8, 7, 6, 5, 4, 3, 2, 1).

Step 3   Tighten your fists as hard as you can. Think about how you feel when you are angry and count to 5.

Step 4   Let your tight fists go and feel the blood rushing down your hands into your arms. It's so pleased that it's no longer being blocked by your tight fists.

Step 5   Now do Steps 3 and 4 three more times very slowly.

Step 6   Sit quietly again and count backwards from 10 again (10, 9, 8, 7, 6, 5, 4, 3, 2, 1) to calm your body down.

You can carry on with this activity on the next sheet (sheet 2.3b)

2.3b Twelve steps (continued)

ACTIVITY   This activity carries on from Sheet 2.3a.

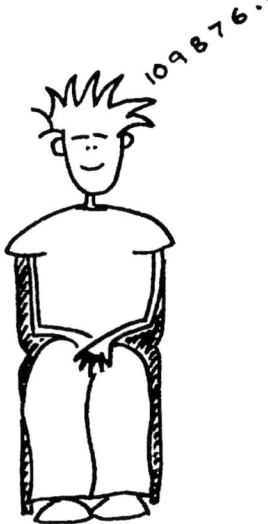

Step 7   Next, lift your shoulders as high as you can. See if your shoulders can touch your ears! You will feel a bit uncomfortable and tight now, but hold on to the tightness and count to 5.

Step 8   Now let go of the tightness in your shoulders. Once again, feel the blood rushing down your neck and into your body. It's so pleased that it's no longer being blocked by your tight shoulders.

Step 9   Do Steps 7 and 8 three more times and then have a rest.

Step 10   Can you draw circles with your elbows? Try one arm at a time, starting with your right arm. First of all, bend your arm so that you touch your shoulder with your right hand. Think of your elbow as a pen and make a circling movement with it, as if you were drawing a circle in the air. Now try this with your left arm. You could then try with both arms together. As you do this, you can almost feel the blood going all round your body.

Step 11   Sit quietly again and count backwards from 10 once more to calm your body down (10, 9, 8, 7, 6, 5, 4, 3, 2, 1).

Step 12   Well done. Now sit quietly for as long as you can, and enjoy feeling calm inside before rushing off to do the next thing.

section 3

Feeling good about yourself

3.1 Who am I?

ACTIVITY   **Thinking about who I am**

In the wheel below, write down things about yourself. First put your name in the middle of the wheel, then write one thing about yourself in each of the spaces (such as, 'I've got curly hair'). You don't need to think too hard about this, just put down the first thing that pops into your head.

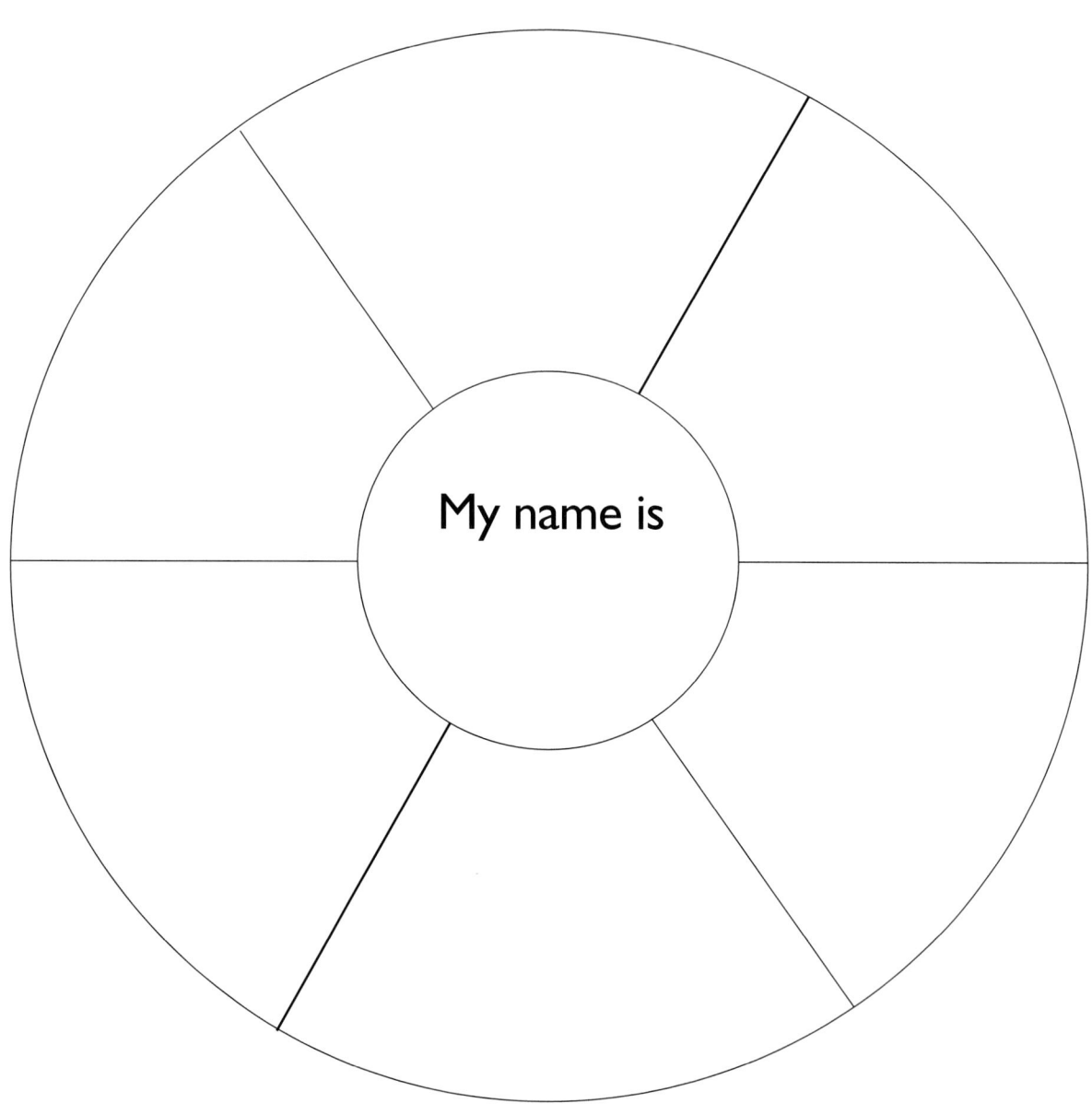

3.2 This is me

NAME: DATE:

ACTIVITY   **My favourite things**
It would be good to know a little more about you. On this sheet, you can tell us about your favourite things.

FAVOURITE **ACTIVITY**

FAVOURITE **FOOD**

FAVOURITE **MUSIC**

FAVOURITE **TV PROGRAMME**

FAVOURITE **CLOTHES**

FAVOURITE **COLOUR**

ACTIVITY   **My good points**
Have fun working out good points about yourself, using as many letters of your first name as possible. For example, if your name is James, it might look like this: (remember, we are only interested in your good points!)

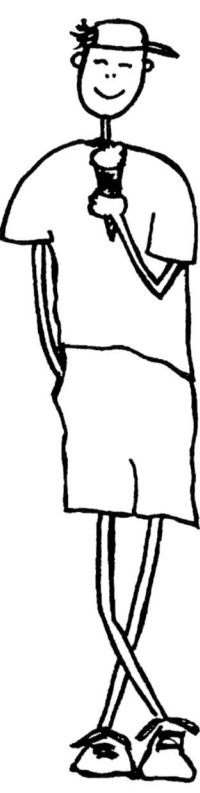

J   Juggles

A   Always tidies up after playing

M   Makes models

E   Enjoys cooking

S   Sings

3.3 All about me

NAME: **DATE:**

ACTIVITY   On this sheet we are going to look at what we can do best. We are also going to think about things we are not so good at and maybe we need help with. There are things that you can help other children with, and it would be useful to know about these too.

Things I do well:

*
*
*
*
*
*

Things I'm not so good at and maybe need help to do:

*
*
*
*
*
*

Things I could help other children do:

*
*
*
*
*
*

3.4 All about my friends

ACTIVITY Let's think about your friends now. Do they look like you, or enjoy doing the same things as you? You could find out by doing the quiz below. Your friends could either be children in the same group as you now, or other children you know.

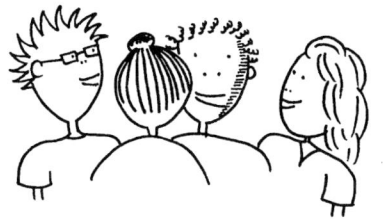

Which of your friends are like you?

Question	My friend called
1. Who is the same age as you?	_____
2. Who has the same colour hair as you?	_____
3. Who has the same colour eyes as you?	_____
4. Who is as tall as you?	_____
5. Who has the same favourite colour as you?	_____
6. Who likes the same TV programme as you?	_____

Now think about the following questions, and add a few of your own

Question	My friend called
1. Who wears glasses?	_____
2. Who has long hair?	_____
3. Who has a baby brother?	_____
4. Who has a sister?	_____
5. Who has a pet cat?	_____
6. Who likes playing football?	_____
7.	_____
8.	_____
9.	_____
10.	_____

3.5 Making new friends

ACTIVITY   When we make new friends, how does it happen? Making and keeping friends is like growing a plant. We keep the plant alive by looking after it. In the same way, we need to take care how we treat our friends (for example, be kind to them). Let's think about how we can do this (brainstorm) and write down our ideas in the leaves below.

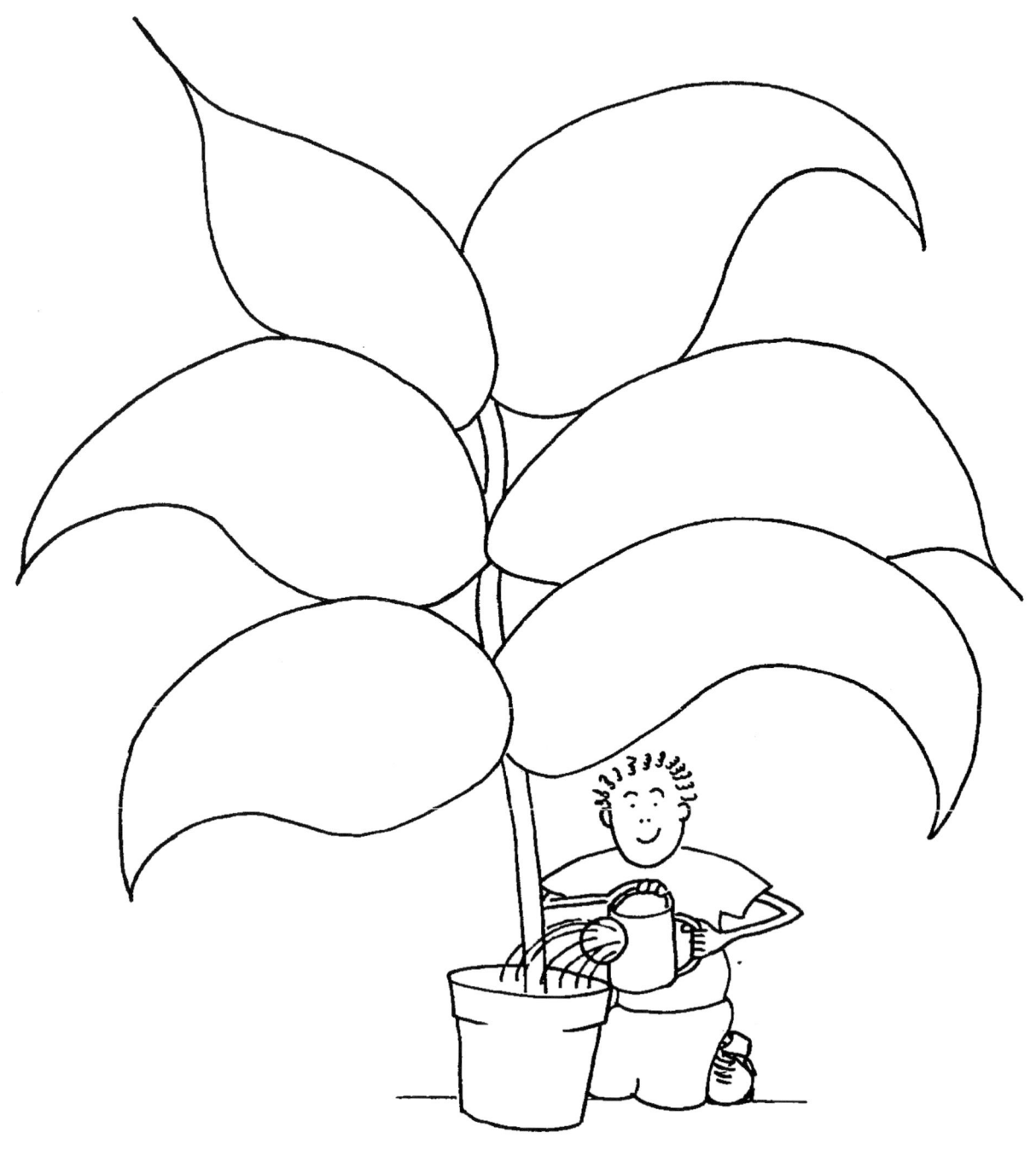

3.6a Getting to know new friends

NAME: DATE:

ACTIVITY We can get to know new friends by talking to them, and asking them questions about themselves. One way we can practise this is by setting up an interview with someone in the group. You may like this interview to be video taped so that you and your friends in the group can watch it later and see how you got on together. You don't need to write down the answers to the questions below, just enjoy talking to each other!

How to set up an interview

Step 1   Divide yourselves into pairs, and call one of each pair A and the other B.

Step 2   Decide whether A or B is going to be the first interviewer.

Step 3   The first interviewer asks their partner questions.

Step 4   Now the other person is the interviewer.

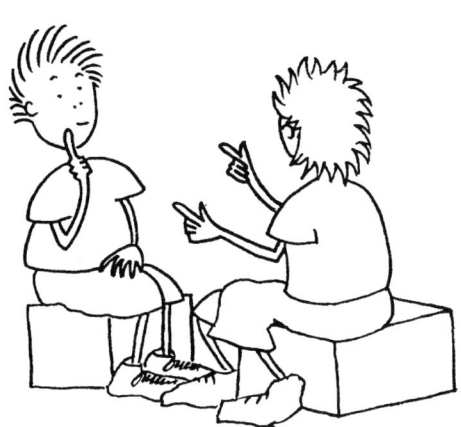

The interview schedule

Name of interviewer	1st:	2nd:
Name of person interviewed	1st:	2nd:

1. How old are you?
2. Do you have any brothers and sisters?
3. Do you have any pets?
4. Where do you live?
5. What school do you go to?
6. What do you like best about school?
7. What is your worst subject at school?
8. What do you enjoy doing most at home?

Now think up two of your own questions to ask your friend (you may like write them down first)

9.

10.

Thank your friend very much for answering these questions

End of interview

3.6b Encouraging self-monitoring (and observation) skills (to be used with Sheet 3.6a)

NAME: DATE:

ACTIVITY When we talk to friends, we use a lot of different skills, such as looking, listening and turn-taking (without interrupting). It is useful to know how much we do these things. If your interview on Sheet 3.6a was videotaped, watch the video now. You could look first at each person in your group as the interviewer and then as the one being interviewed. As you watch the video, use the following symbols to show how well you think each person did in this activity.

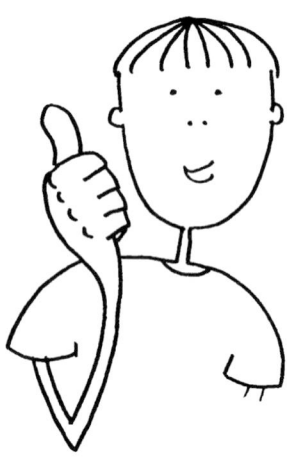

Symbols to use when filling in the table below:

✓ good
? needs a bit of help here
✗ not very good

Name of inter-viewer or person interviewed	Were they looking at the other person?	Were they listening to the other person?	Were they taking turns?	Did you notice anything else? (e.g. speaking out)

3.7 Prouding on a daily basis

If we stop and think, there are so many things we can feel proud about. It is important to know this, and to write down something you are proud of. It may be something you said or did, or something you have been working on for a long time. You may be proud of making a new friend. You can start by thinking of it right now! Let's call this 'Prouding Time'.

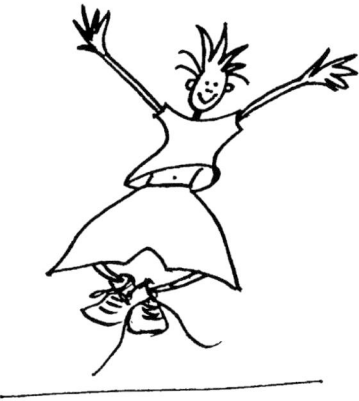

Day	Today, I'm proud of...
Monday	
Tuesday	
Wednesday	
Thursday	
Friday	
Saturday	
Sunday	

section 4

Getting out of difficulties (e.g. teasing and bullying)

4.1 Looking at feelings we like and don't like

It's useful to look at feelings we like and don't like, because that way we can understand ourselves better. If we know what feelings we don't like, we can try to work out why and then do something about it.

NAME: DATE:

ACTIVITY   Let's start by thinking about the feelings we like and write them down in the first box below. We can then write down the feelings we don't like in the second box next to it.

Feelings we like
1.
2.
3.
4.
5.
6.
7.
8.

Feelings we don't like
1.
2.
3.
4.
5.
6.
7.
8.

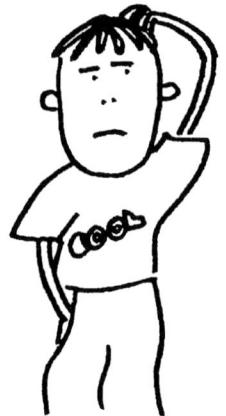

4.2 What makes us have feelings we don't like?

Sometimes we have feelings we don't like when something happens that makes us feel uncomfortable. Let's think a bit more about these feelings now.

NAME: DATE:

ACTIVITY If you did the activity on Sheet 4.1, copy the feelings you wrote down in the second box into the box called 'Feelings we don't like' below. When you have done that, think about what makes you feel this way. For example, feeling tired may be a feeling you don't like, and going to bed late may make you feel this way

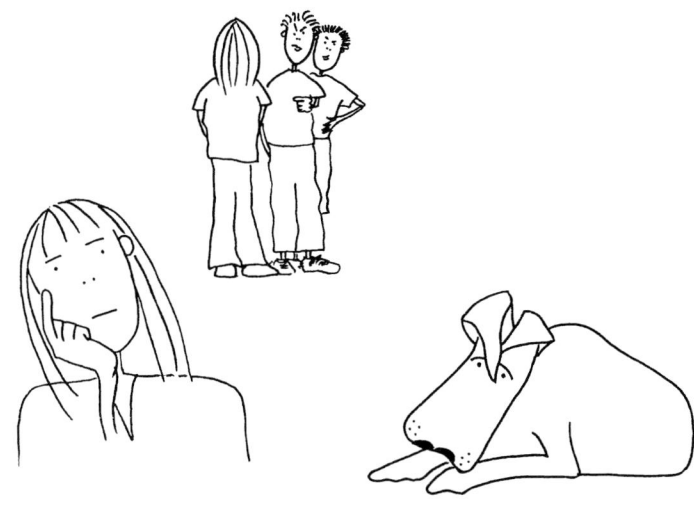

Feelings we don't like		What makes us feel this way?
1.	→	1.
2.	→	2.
3.	→	3.
4.	→	4.
5.	→	5.
6.	→	6.
7.	→	7.
8.	→	8.

Do you agree that when we are teased or bullied we feel scared, sad and lonely? Let's see what we can do about these feelings we don't like.

4.3 Taking a closer look at teasing and bullying

NAME: DATE:

ACTIVITY If we think more about what happened and why we were teased or bullied, we can work out what to do about it. A good way to start is to try and fill in the table below. Don't worry if you don't know the answer or can't remember what happened exactly, just have a go and see how far you get. Remember all that you write down is private to you, so you can choose who else sees it.

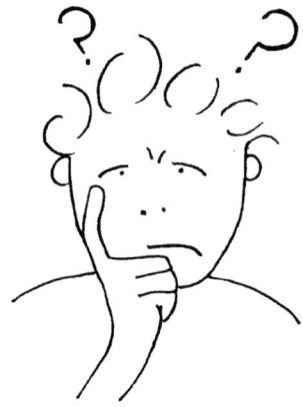

Date it happened	
What time did it happen?	
Where did it happen?	
What happened?	
How did it happen?	
Who did it?	
Why did it happen?	

4.4 What do **YOU** do when teased or bullied?

NAME: DATE:

ACTIVITY   What do YOU do when you are teased or
bullied, and do you think it helps? Spend a few
moments thinking about this and then write
down what you do.

When I am teased or bullied I usually . . .

What happens next?

Do you think that what you do is helpful?

4.5 Helpful and unhelpful ways of dealing with teasing and bullying

There are helpful and unhelpful ways of dealing with teasing and bullying. We are going to look at these now, so that we can decide what might be the best way for you. One way of deciding whether what we are doing is helpful or unhelpful, is to look at what happens next. For example, if you hit the bully back and then get into trouble with the teacher, is hitting a useful way of behaving?

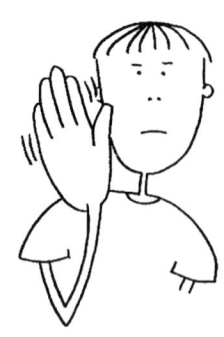

NAME: DATE:

ACTIVITY   Look at what other children have said about what they do about teasing and bullying. Do you agree with them?

Helpful ways		What do you think happens next?
Ignore it and walk away (turn away and run if necessary)	→	
Say 'No' firmly and walk away	→	
Make it into a joke (humour helps)	→	
Think about what you are good at and be proud of it	→	
Tell the teacher and/or an adult you know (such as a parent)	→	
Make friends with the bullies	→	

Now think about unhelpful ways of dealing with teasing and bullying.

Unhelpful ways		What do you think happens next?
Arguing with the bully	→	
Hitting the bully	→	

4.6 What can **YOU** do about being teased and bullied?

How can we change the scared, sad and lonely feelings we have when we are being teased and bullied? One way is by thinking about teasing and bullying in a different way. We can do this by imagining that when we are teased or bullied, we put on a special cape that protects us from the horrible things that are happening to us.

NAME: DATE:

ACTIVITY   You could practise putting on this imaginary protective cape in your group, in three steps.

Step 1   Everyone in the group makes a paper dart, and writes on the dart all the horrible things that have been said or done to them by the bullies.

Step 2   Next, take turns in your group to put on the imaginary protective cape. You could use a dustbin bag for this, by cutting out holes for arms and head and putting it on (not everyone may want to do this).

Step 3   The person with the special cape on stands in the middle of a circle, and the rest of the children in the group throw the paper darts at the person wearing the protective cape.

You'll see that the darts just fall off, they don't tear or pierce the cape (dustbin bag) in any way, so they can't really hurt the person inside. This activity shows that if we can think of horrible words as puffs of air which turn into nothing, they don't have to go inside and hurt us and make us feel scared, sad and lonely.

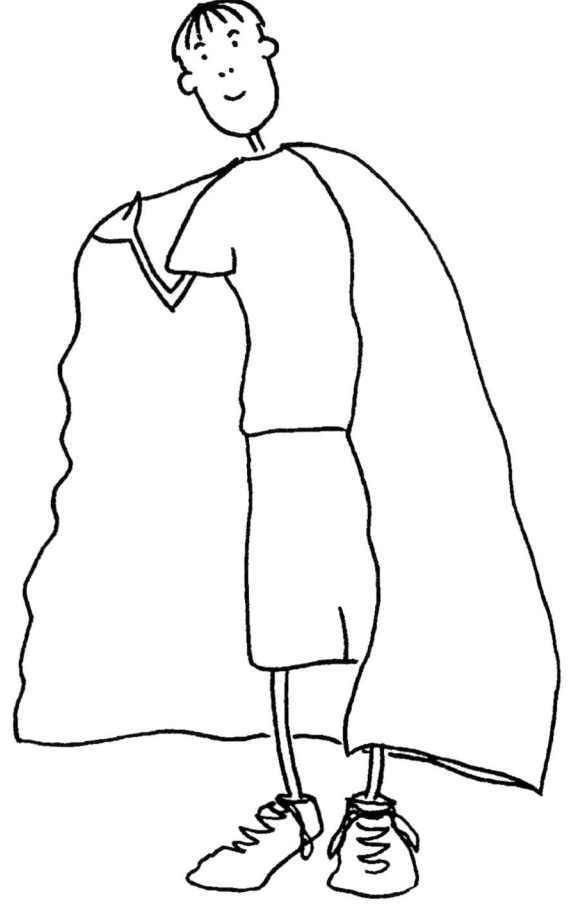

4.7 Putting on your protective cape

If you completed Sheet 4.6, you will remember that we looked at how putting on your protective cape can help when something happens that makes you feel uncomfortable. We are going to practise this again now.

NAME: DATE:

ACTIVITY   Imagine putting on your protective cape, and then remind yourself that when something happens that makes you feel uncomfortable, it is helpful to keep calm, to think about something that you like or that makes you feel good, and to get on with other things. If you did Sheet 4.3, you could look again at the things you wrote in the table, and remember what happened. Only this time, you are wearing your protective cape to help you with the uncomfortable feelings.

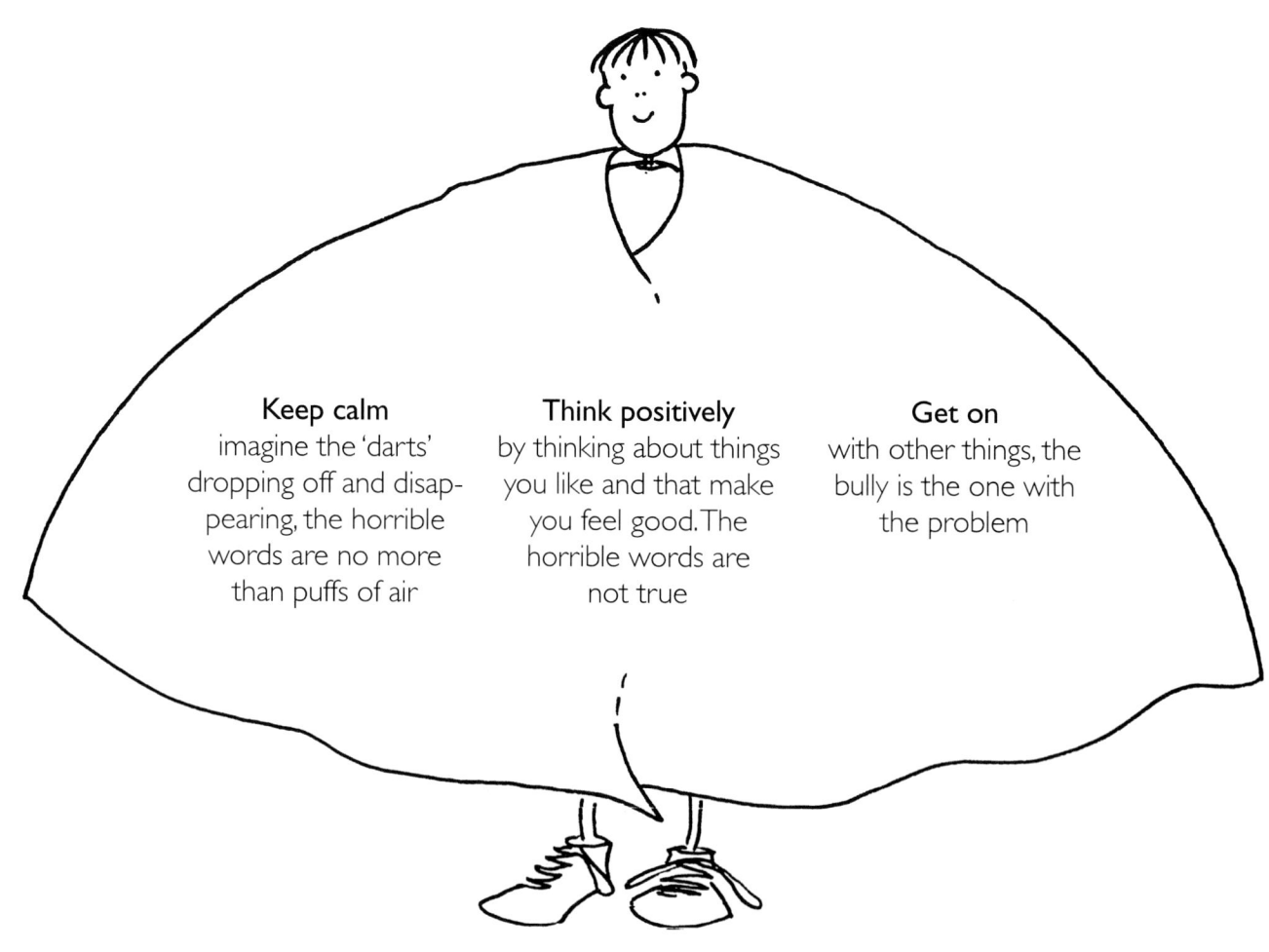

Keep calm
imagine the 'darts' dropping off and disappearing, the horrible words are no more than puffs of air

Think positively
by thinking about things you like and that make you feel good. The horrible words are not true

Get on
with other things, the bully is the one with the problem

4.8 Remember ACT for fast action in difficult situations

When we find ourselves in difficult and uncomfortable situations, it can be very helpful to have a special code word that helps us to remember what to do.

NAME: DATE:

ACTIVITY Let's crack the special code word now and then you can remember to use it when you feel uncomfortable about what is happening.

TODAY'S MISSION To crack the special code

REASON FOR NEEDING SPECIAL CODE WORD To help out in difficult situations

REASON ACCEPTED Please attend carefully, as special code word is about to be revealed

YOUR SPECIAL CODE WORD   =   ACT

Please listen carefully for instructions on how to crack the special code word

A	AVOID getting involved
C	COPE by keeping calm
T	TELL someone (perhaps a teacher or parent)

YOUR NEXT MISSION   =   To learn the special code word

To accomplish this mission you will need to look at the box above for 1 minute. Now cover up the box containing the special code word with a piece of paper and fill in the box below:

A	
C	
T	

Well done, for successfully accomplishing this mission!

---

section 5

How your voice works

5.1 Feeling your voice buzzing

We use our voice every day, talking, singing, laughing and shouting, but how often do we think about it and just how it works?

NAME: DATE:

ACTIVITY   **Feeling your voice buzzing**
Put your finger tips on your throat. Do you know the place called the 'Adam's apple'? This is where the voice box (larynx) is housed in your throat. Men and older boys have a bigger 'Adam's apple', so it is easier to feel.

Now that you have found the right place, with your lips closed make a humming sound. You will feel the buzz in your finger tips. You can also feel the buzz in your lips and on your nose. Do this several times. Feel all the buzzing places: larynx, nose and lips.

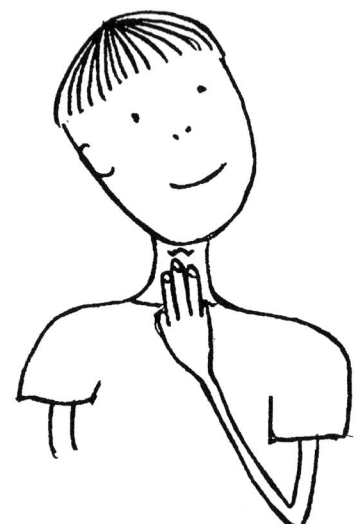

- The sound /**m**/* is made with air coming down the nose, that's why it makes a lot of buzz. /**n**/ and /**ng**/ sounds are also made in the nose.
- /**m**/, /**n**/ and /ng/ are the three nasal sounds in English. /**ng**/ comes only in the middle or at the end of a word.

ACTIVITY   **Thinking and writing**
Can you add some more words with nasal sounds?

meal   hammer   shame

neck   funny   fun

            finger   sing

*When a letter is shown between two slashes like this (//), it means the sound not the letter written. For example, in the word 'photo' the first sound is /f/, although from the spelling of the word you might think it is /p/.

5.2 What makes the buzz of the voice?

NAME: DATE:

ACTIVITY The voice is made in a little box in the throat, called the voice box or larynx. In the box there are two very precious little bands (vocal folds), which can come together. When they come close together and air passes between them they move very quickly (vibrate), making a tiny sound. The air used for voice comes from the lungs. We need air to breathe to keep alive but we also need air to make sounds in speaking.

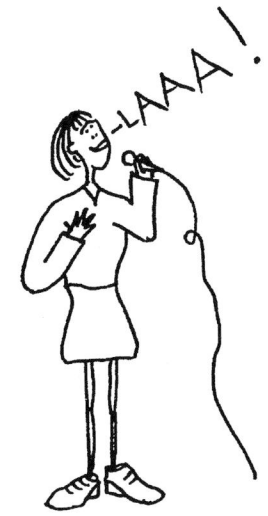

ACTIVITY

-LAAA!

VOICE BOX → ◁▷ ← VOICE BANDS

WIND PIPES →

LUNGS SENDING UP AIR

- The picture shows how air travels up from the lungs into the windpipe and through the voice box.
- A tiny sound is made as air passes between the bands.
- The tiny sound gets bigger as it goes on its journey, into the mouth and out through the lips.

Can you follow the journey? Take a coloured pen and draw how the air travels up from the lungs and out through the lips.

5.3 Using your voice in different ways

NAME: DATE:

The little sound the voice box makes with the bands is so precious, just like a jewel, and we need to take care of it.

The tiniest sound used for talking, which doesn't have any voice at all, is WHISPER. We whisper a secret or a joke to just one other person, when we don't want anyone else to hear. Some sounds, such as /p/t/s/f/, are just whispers and are called VOICELESS CONSONANTS.

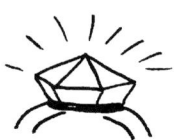

ACTIVITY **Doing and checking**
- Whisper something to someone near to you (no, not in a lesson!). Choose a time when you are alone with someone. Give your message very, very quietly – no voice.
- Did they understand what you said? If not, do you know why that was?

When we are talking to someone else, but not in secret, we need to talk a bit louder. We can call this 'TALKING BETWEEN TWO PEOPLE', because it's only one other person who needs to hear.

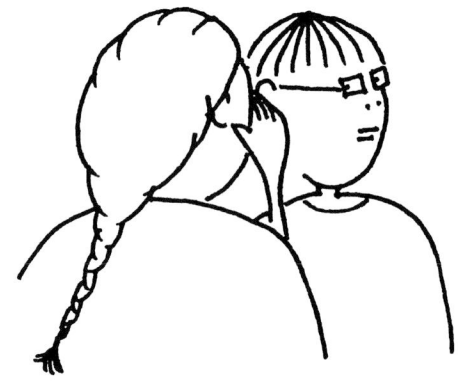

ACTIVITY **Think and write**
Make a list of people you talk to in this way.

5.4 Taking care of your voice

If we're talking to a few people, perhaps round a table at home or at school, we need to use a little bit more voice – how about calling this 'TALKING ROUND THE TABLE'.

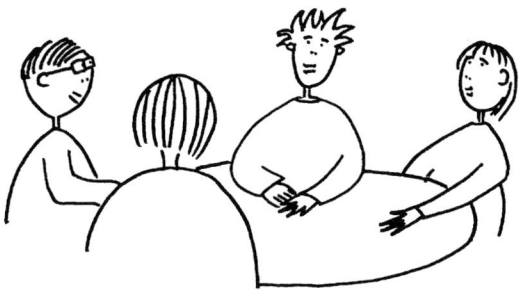

ACTIVITY   Think and write

Make a list of the ways you talk to a small group of people: for example, 'having a chat with some friends'. You can make this list gradually, as you begin to notice more about the way you use your voice at different times.

When you speak out in class to a big group, you need to open your mouth well to let out all the sound.

- You need to go slowly so that everyone can follow.
- You need to make all the consonants as clearly as you can.
- You do not need to shout – that will hurt those precious bands.
- If you shout too much it will make your voice hoarse and husky.
- If your voice is hoarse, it is more difficult for other people to understand you.
- To describe the kind of voice we need to use when we talk to a group of people – we could call it 'WIDER VOICE'.

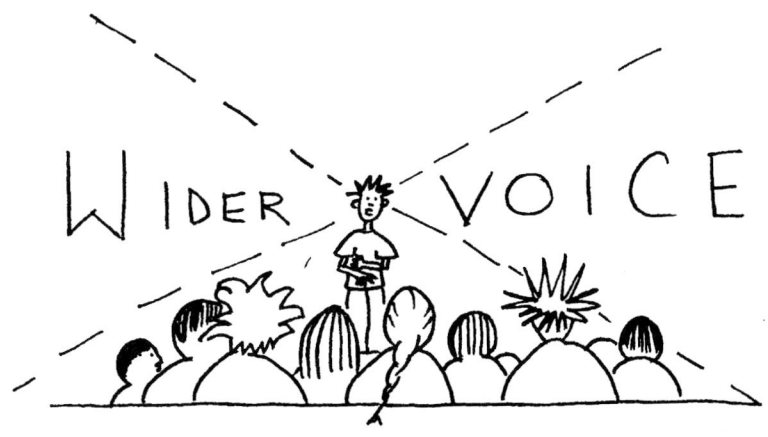

ACTIVITY   Thinking and deciding

What do you think about the name 'WIDER VOICE'? Perhaps you would like to choose another name. You can call it whatever you like, if it helps you to remember.

5.5a Making your own voice bugle and your daily voice diary

NAME: DATE:

Look at the picture on Sheet 5.5b. This gives a picture of the ways the voice can work – gradually getting wider from just a whisper, through the ways we have thought about, right up to a shout. How about making a voice bugle of your own? You could add pictures and words of your own that help you to remember it.

* * * * * * * * DANGER ZONE * * * * * *

Look at the end of the voice bugle – you are now entering a danger zone. Remember the two words SHOUTING and DANGER. Some kinds of shouting hurt those precious bands in the voice box, and may really damage them so that you will have a hoarse voice all the time – that won't help you to speak out clearly.

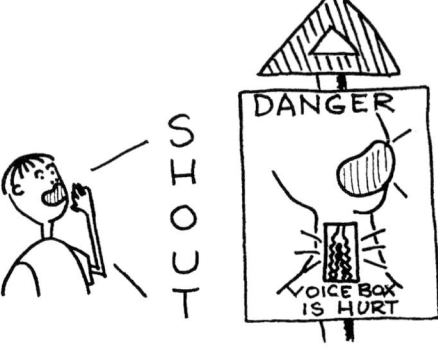

ACTIVITY Your daily voice diary

At the end of each day (over a week), try to think how you've used your voice. Decide if you've used your voice in the right way for what is happening at the time. Did you shout a secret? You can use this chart to keep your diary, but if you like you can make a chart of your own. You can fill in most of the columns with just yes or no answers.

Date	How many people were there?	Did they understand you?	Did you speak too quietly?	Did you speak too loudly?	Was the volume just right?	Did you speak too slowly or too quickly?

NAME: DATE:

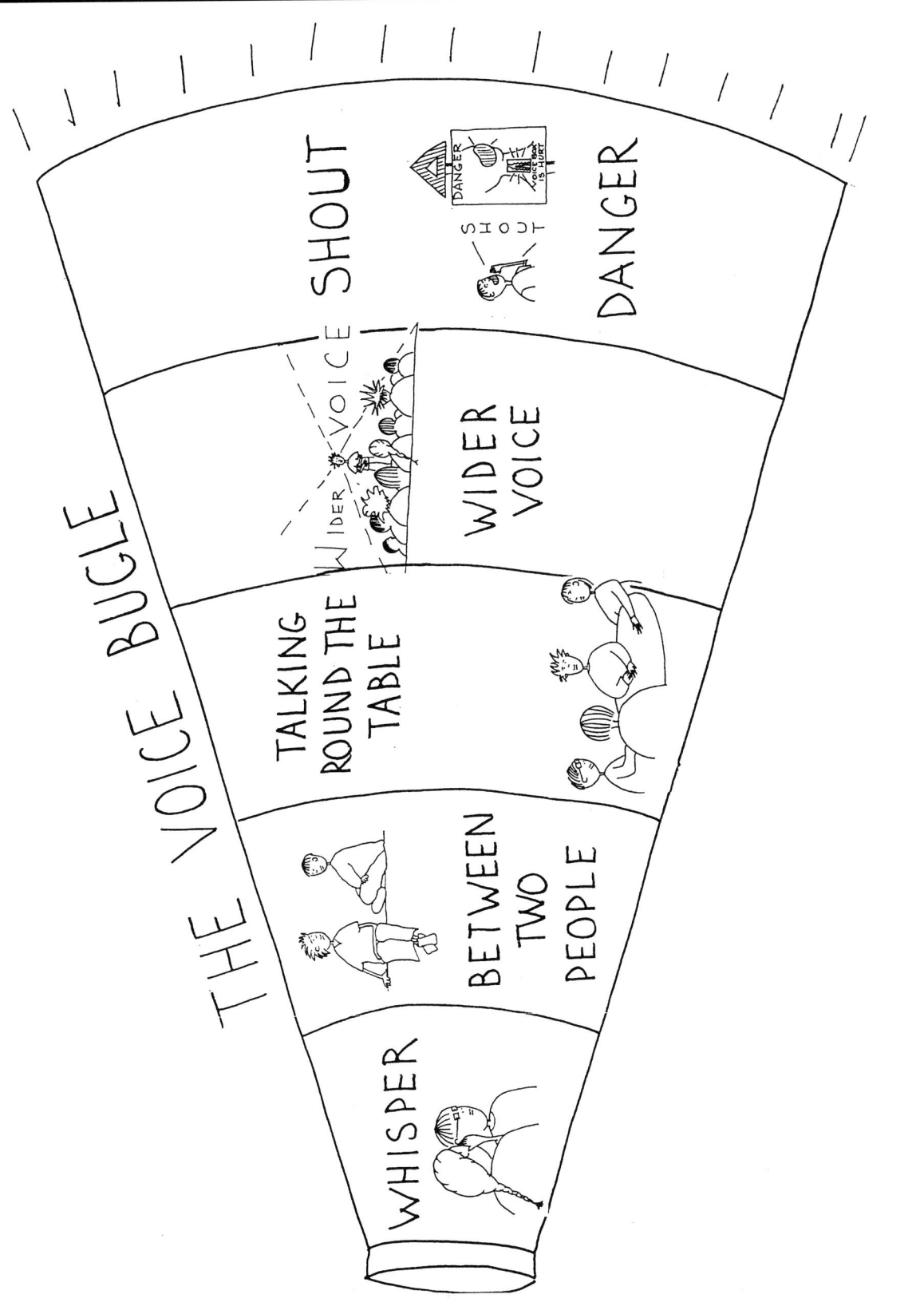

THE VOICE BUGLE

WHISPER

BETWEEN TWO PEOPLE

TALKING ROUND THE TABLE

WIDER VOICE

SHOUT

DANGER

NAME: DATE:

A few tips
- When speaking to one other person, be sure to be close enough to them so that you do not need to shout.
- When there is a vowel sound at the start of a word, be sure to start off gently.
- Try to be relaxed when speaking, keep your shoulders down and open your mouth well in a relaxed way.
- Coughing and throat clearing will irritate your vocal folds and throat, so try not to do it – if you feel like clearing your throat, try a good hard swallow instead.
- If you have a cold or cough, drink plenty of water.
- Always drink plenty of water, but try to avoid pop and fizzy drinks.
- Avoid talking in noisy places like discos.
- Avoid shouting, especially in the open air.
- Don't start smoking – if you have already done so, stop! Smoking is very damaging for your throat and voice, and has long-term dangers for you. How would it affect your lungs – vital for breathing and speaking?
- Try not to speak for too long on one breath – your voice will begin to fade and you'll feel seriously out of breath. You will also get very tense, with trying to push out the last little bit of air.
- Imagine your voice is being made in your head, rather than in your throat.
- If you have a sore or aching throat for any reason, don't ignore it – your voice box is telling you to take special care. Never force your voice.
- There may be times when you will really need to rest your voice – that may mean not speaking at all for some hours.

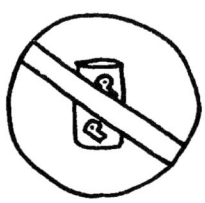

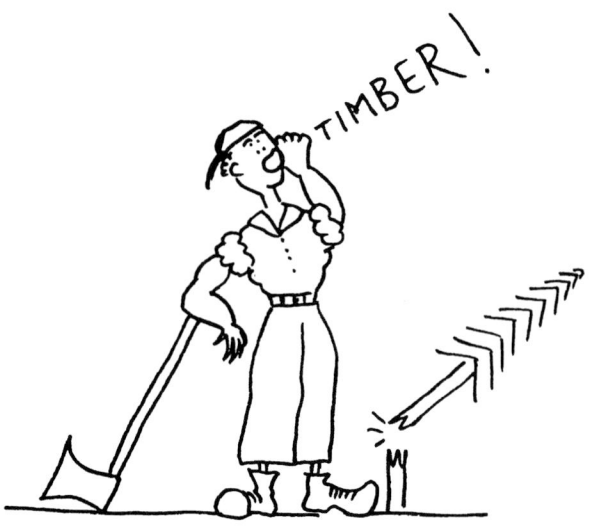

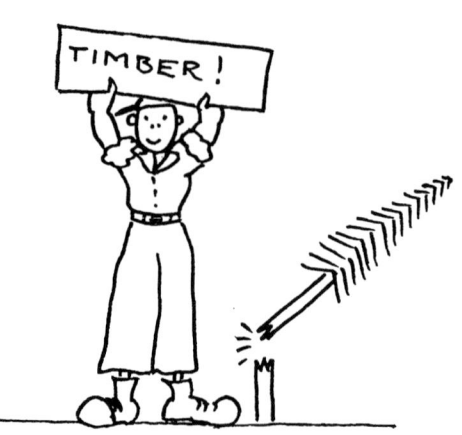

section 6

Sending messages through speaking

6.1 Sending messages through speaking

NAME: DATE:

There are lots of ways to send messages to other people, such as writing, signing or email. You will be able to think of some more. One of the most important ways of sending messages is through speaking. You can use speech either on the phone or through a video or tape recorder. You can speak directly to one other person, to a few people or to lots of people. You can use speech to say how you feel, to say what you want, to tell a story, to ask a question, to give an answer, to try out new ideas, and to make a joke.

How the body speaks

So that other people can understand us when we speak, we need to make speech sounds clearly. For some people this may be difficult and it helps to understand how and where speech sounds are made. We need five main parts of our body to be able to speak:

1.   the ears
2.   the brain
3.   the lungs and the windpipe (trachea)
4.   the throat and the voice box (larynx)
5.   the mouth

This is what happens

- The ears hear the speech sounds, words and messages coming in.
- The brain understands what is being said.
- The brain decides what we want to say.
- Air is sent up from the lungs.
- Small voice sounds are made in the throat.
- Air and sounds travel further up the throat and are directed into the mouth or nose (only a few sounds are made in the nose).
- In the mouth the tongue and lips move to produce all sorts of sounds.
- The brain is kept busy sending messages to organise and control all the complicated movements that are needed for talking.

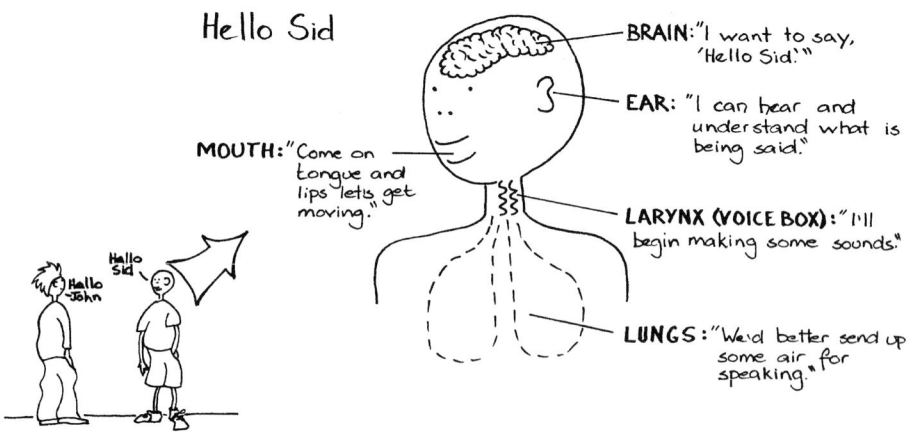

ACTIVITY   Thinking and writing

Make a list of all the sounds in speech that you can think of – watch out, not all of them are the same in writing! Try thinking of the sounds in your own name first.

Put your sound list here:

6.2 The sounds in our language

NAME: DATE:

What is the name of the language you usually use? Can you list some of the sounds from that language?

ACTIVITY **Asking others**

Perhaps there are some children in your group who speak a different language from your own. See if they will say some of the different sounds for you. Sounds are divided up into vowels and consonants. For now, we will look at the English sounds.

Vowels

- a e i o u – this is how vowels appear in writing.
- All words have a vowel sound and this part of the word is usually fairly easy to make.
- In speaking, vowels often come together, or next to other sounds which change the way we say them. They become like two vowels together, and are called diphthongs. The words 'my' and 'I' sound the same but are written differently. Words such as 'hit' are spelt with the same letter 'i', but sound quite different.
- When we make a vowel or a diphthong, the small sound made in the voice box travels up the throat to the mouth, getting stronger.
- The mouth changes shape and makes the sounds change.

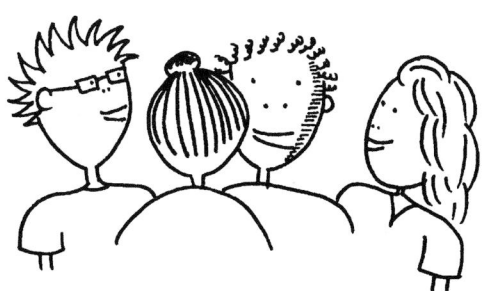

ACTIVITY **Feeling your voice buzz**

Put three fingers in front of your throat and gently touch the middle (harder and sensitive) part. Say 'ah' – can you feel the buzz in your fingers? You may have to move your fingers to find the place where you can feel it. Ask someone else to say 'ah', and you feel the buzz in their throat. Now see what happens when you blow – is there a buzz?

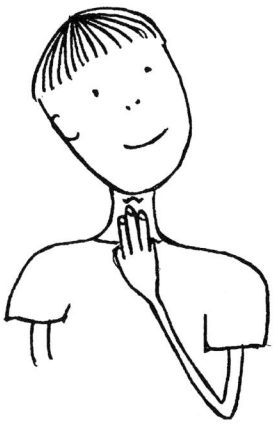

- The buzz is the movement of the vocal folds in the voice box as air passes through them. All vowels are made with the vocal folds vibrating, so all vowels are voiced sounds.

6.3 Consonants

Look at the list of sounds you made for the activity on Sheet 6.1. Did you list all the VOWELS? All the other sounds you listed that are not vowels, are CONSONANTS. We need to know a lot about consonants because they are so important in allowing the message we are sending to be understood by the person or group of people receiving it. We all know what it feels like not to be understood.

- Sometimes we are not understood because we have spoken too quickly or too quietly.
- Sometimes we are not understood because the consonant has not been said clearly or has been missed out.
- Some consonants are complicated and may be difficult to produce clearly.
- If we can learn more about the way consonants are made, it will help us to make them clearly.
- We need to know which parts of the mouth are used and how the sounds are made.
- We need to be able to tell if the voice is making a buzzing sound or not.

A picture of the mouth

In the mouth, the small sounds of voice and air coming up from the lungs and through the voice box, are worked on to make them into recognisable vowels and consonants. Here is a picture of the mouth. Can you believe how many fast and complicated movements it can make? There may be some words in the picture that you haven't seen before. They will help you later.

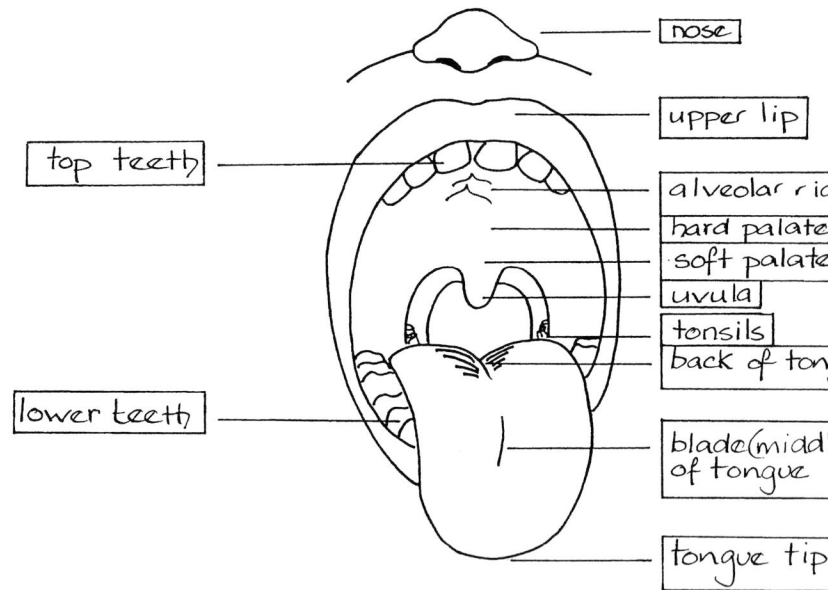

- When we learn to make sounds, it is really helpful to be sure about which part of our mouth is being used. You will see later that we use more than one part of the mouth to make a sound.
- Parts of the mouth are fixed and do not move, such as the teeth and the hard palate. Other parts move, such as the tongue and the lips.

6.4a Which parts of the mouth do we use for consonants?

NAME: DATE:

ACTIVITY   Take a sheet of paper, or use the other side of this sheet. Sit down in front of a mirror – a big one, if you have one at home or school. Draw a picture of your own mouth, then use the picture on Sheet 6.3 to label the parts. If you don't want to draw your own mouth, ask someone else at home or at school to let you draw theirs. Whoever you draw, you'll find that the mouth is not the same as the picture here. This is because each person is different and special. Some people have a shorter tongue or gaps in their teeth. If we all looked the same, how would we know who was who?

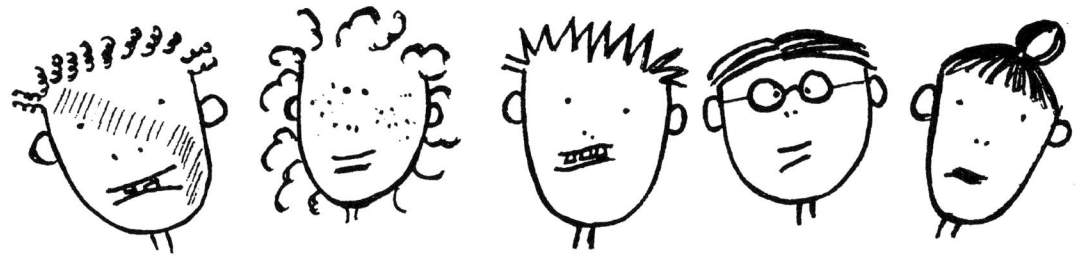

ACTIVITY   **Saying and thinking**
Say the sounds in the table below. After saying each one, write beside it which two parts of the mouth you think that you are using. You may need to use some of the new words shown in the picture of the mouth on Sheet 6.3.

- It's really important that you write down what you think you are doing, so don't ask anyone else to tell you. If you're not sure, put a tick in the 'Not sure' column below.
- It doesn't matter if someone else does it in a different way, or you are not sure of the answers – we will be learning more about all the sounds later on.

Sound	Parts of the mouth used in making sound		
	1st part	2nd part	Not sure (tick)
/f/			
/m/			
/l/			
/d/			

6.4b Sound chart

NAME: DATE:

Lists of consonants and where they are made

Sounds are made with two parts of the mouth, usually one moving part and one fixed part. The sound chart below shows which mouth parts are used for each consonant. There is another chart on sheet 6.4c to use for sounds in languages other than English.

Sound					
Both lips (bilabial)	Upper teeth to lower lip (labiodental)	Tongue tip to alveolar ridge (alveolar)	Tongue to front of hard palate (post-alveolar)	Tongue to palate (palato-alveolar)	Back of tongue to back of palate (velar)
p b m w	f v	t d n l r s z **Tongue tip to teeth (Dental)** th <u>th</u>	sh ʒ	ch j	k g
Column 1	Column 2	Column 3	Column 4	Column 5	Column 6

6.4c Chart for sounds other than English

NAME: DATE:

Do you speak any languages other than English? If you do, you could use this chart to think about where the sounds in that language are made. If you know even more languages, your helper could photocopy this chart so that you have a sound chart for each of the languages you know!

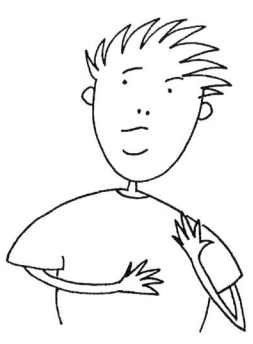

	Bilabial (both lips)	Labio-dental (tongue and teeth)	Dental (teeth)	Alveolar (behind top teeth)	Post-alveolar (behind alveolar)	Retroflex (tongue tip back)	Palatal (tongue to hard palate)	Velar (tongue to soft palate)	Uvular (tongue to uvula)	Pharyngeal (sounds in throat)	Glottal (with voice bands)
Plosive										▓	
Nasal										▓	▓
Trill											▓
Tap or flap								▓			▓
Fricative								▓			
Lateral fricative	▓									▓	▓
Approximant											▓
Lateral approximant	▓									▓	▓

6.5　Lip sounds: /p/b/m/w/

NAME:　　　　　　　　　　　　　　　　　　DATE:

If you look at column 1 on the sound chart on Sheet 6.4b, you will see four sounds listed under 'Both lips': they are /p/b/m/w/.

ACTIVITY　**Listening and watching**

Get someone (at home or at school) to do this with you. Ask your helper to say each of the sounds. You will notice that some of the sounds are long (/**m**/ and /**w**/) and some of them are short (/**p**/ and /**b**/).

Ask your helper to say each of the sounds while you watch their lips and listen. The helper must be very careful not to say the name of the letter, but just to say the sound.

- In /m/ the lips press together and the voice box vibrates to make a buzzing sound, in words such as **m**ay, ar**m**, hu**mm**ing and ar**m**our. You will feel a buzz in your throat and on your lips.
- In /w/ the lips make a round shape but don't quite touch, and then move apart, in words such as **w**ay, mo**w**er and ho**w**.

Question: (tick your answer)　　　　　　Yes　　　　No　　　　Nearly

Can you make the sound /**m**/?
(just put your lips together and hum)

Can you make the sound /**w**/?
(push your lips forward)

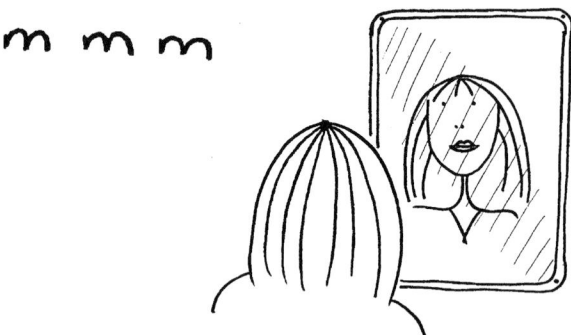

ACTIVITY　**Thinking and writing**

List four words beginning with /**m**/ and four words beginning with /**w**/. (You could use a dictionary if you like, but have a try on your own first, or ask someone to help you.) Write your words down here:

Words beginning with /**m**/　　　　　　　　Words beginning with /**w**/
- 　　　　　　　　　　　　　　　　　　　-
- 　　　　　　　　　　　　　　　　　　　-
- 　　　　　　　　　　　　　　　　　　　-
- 　　　　　　　　　　　　　　　　　　　-

6.6 The difference between /p/ and /b/

NAME: DATE:

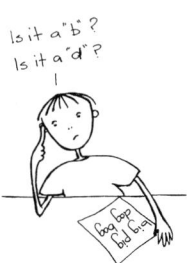

Don't these two letters, 'p' and 'b', look alike! We need to be careful that we write them the right way up and the right way round. If the letters are the wrong way up, we can't be sure what the word says. Is it big or pig, dog or bog? It is the same in speaking – we need to make a difference between /p/ and /b/ so that other people know exactly what we are saying: 'Give me the pea', not 'Give me the bee'.

- For both /p/ and /b/ sounds the lips move in the same way – so how are the two sounds different? The clue is the buzz made in the voice box.

ACTIVITY   Listening and feeling

Ask someone at home or at school to do this with you. Get your speech and language therapist or your teacher to practise it with you first.
- Put your fingers on the throat of your helper and ask them to say these two words: la**b** la**p**
- Can you feel a difference in your fingers at the end of the words?
- One sound had a finger buzz at the end and the other did not.

Listen and feel, and decide which word had the buzz.
- /**b**/ has a buzz – it is called a voiced consonant.
- /**p**/ does not have a buzz – it is called a voiceless consonant.

Ask your helper to say the words again – this time, when you feel the buzz with your fingers on their throat, get them to repeat the end sound, so that you can listen carefully and feel:

     lab – b b b   lap – p p p

The p p p comes with a burst of air – feel that by asking your helper to say the /p/ against the back of your hand.

Can you think of some other words in pairs which end with /**p**/ or /**b**/? You and your helper could think of them together – write them down here, then get your helper to say them while you listen and feel. Always listen carefully when other people speak to you. Try to notice how they make **a** /**p**/ or a /**b**/ sound.

ACTIVITY   Listening and recognising sounds in **different** positions

Ask someone at home or at school to read the following words to you in any order (but try not to look at them!). You decide which box each word should go in, the 'buzz' box or the 'no buzz' box, and write it in.

ball, robe, rope, harbour, cup, baby, pipe, bad, speak, shepherd, armband, cupboard

/b/ buzz
/p/ no buzz

6.7 Lips, teeth and tongue sounds

NAME: DATE:

Find your sound chart (Sheet 6.4b), and look at the list in column 2. /f/ and /v/ are two sounds that are made by putting top teeth against lower lip, and sending out a long stream of air. They are both long sounds:

$$/f \longrightarrow / \qquad\qquad /v \longrightarrow /$$

How are they different? Perhaps you already know the answer. Just to make sure, try this listening game.

ACTIVITY   Listening

Ask your helper at home or at school to say the words on the list. Listen and put a tick under the 'buzz' heading if you think you hear a buzz on those upper teeth to lower lip sounds:

	No buzz	Buzz		No buzz	Buzz
four			laugh		
coughing			oven		
love			value		
half			offer		

Upper teeth to lower lip
Feel air on lower lip

You will have noticed that the /f/ sound is not always spelt with an 'f' letter!

Now look at the bottom of column 3 of your sound chart. /th/ is written twice, which means there are two sounds, but they are written with the same letters. We have to listen really carefully to hear the difference. To make these two sounds, the tongue tip is placed just behind or just through the top teeth. If you don't have any front teeth or you have gaps at the front of your mouth, it will be easy to see your tongue coming forward. (All children lose their teeth at some time – these are the first, baby teeth, and they come out to make space for the second teeth.)

So /th/ is written twice because there are two different consonants that sound almost the same. They are found in words such as 'think' and 'then'. In 'think', it is just the sound of air blowing between tongue and teeth. For the /th/ in 'then', you can hear and feel a buzz – it is a VOICED CONSONANT. It may help you to remember if we put a line under the voiced /th/, like this, /<u>th</u>/ to show that it has the voice buzz.

ACTIVITY   Listening

Ask someone to do this with you, at home or at school. Ask your helper to say these words. Decide if the consonant is made with a buzz (/<u>th</u>/) or without a buzz (/th/), then tick the right box.

	bath	thunder	them
Buzz			
No buzz			

6.8 The long consonants: /f/th/<u>th</u>/

NAME: DATE:

ACTIVITY **Looking**

Use a hand mirror to look at the front of your mouth. Smile, and now answer the questions below (tick 'Yes' or 'No').

	Yes	No
Have you still got your front teeth?		
Have you got a gap at the front?		
If you have a gap, can you see the new teeth coming?		
Have you got your new teeth already?		

ACTIVITY **Listening**

We need to listen carefully to hear the difference between /f/ and /th/ – the no buzz (voiceless) sounds. It does not matter if you have not learnt to say them yet. Some people never use /th/ when they speak, so it's not a very important sound.

Ask someone at home or at school to do this with you. Get your helper to read the words in any order. Watch their face carefully, and tick the box when they say a word with /th/ or /f/. For /th/ you will see their tongue, and for /f/ you will see their teeth on their lower lip.

	/th/	/f/
thumb		
moth		
fun		
think		
both		
fork		
fin		
thin		
four		
three		
laugh (Remember that sometimes the sound is spelt completely differently.)		

If you can manage these, ask your helper to say the words again while they hold a sheet of paper in front of their mouth, so you can't see if their tongue is showing. You'll need to listen very carefully. Some people find it very difficult to hear the difference between these two sounds, but we usually know which word it is in a sentence because of the meaning.

Put tongue gently between teeth

Feel air between tongue and teeth

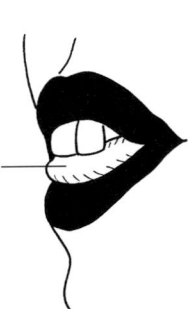

6.9 Some air sounds: /p/f/th/

NAME: DATE:

Three of the consonant sounds you already know about are easy to spot, because you can feel the air as it pops or streams out through your mouth. These three consonant sounds are /p/f/th/. These three sounds do not have a voice buzz with them. Air comes up from the lungs, passes through the voice box without making a sound, and on into the mouth where the mouth makes some changes:

- for /th/ the air pushes its way between the tongue and the teeth to make a long sound /th——►/
- for /f/ the air pushes out between the upper teeth and lower lip to make a long sound /f——►/
- for /p/ the air pops out by bursting open the lips, to make a short sound – /pppppp/.

ACTIVITY **Listening and feeling**

Ask someone at home or at school to do this with you. Get your helper to sit opposite to you. Give them one of your hands to hold up to their mouth. Then they gently whisper:

- /p/   /p/   /p/ (short sounds)
- /th/ (long sound)
- /f/ (long sound)

Feel each stream of air on the back of your hand. It's a help to listen carefully as well as to feel the air. Make sure your helper doesn't put a buzz into any of the sounds. Would you like to have a try at saying the sounds now, while your helper feels the air on the back of their hand? If you manage to do this, feel the air on the back of your own hand as you make the sounds.

Questions (tick one of the boxes)

	Yes	No	Nearly
Did you manage to whisper the sounds?			
Did you manage /ppp/ in a whisper?			
Did you manage the long /f ——► /?			
Did you manage the long /th ——► /?			

Which sound did you like making best? (tick the box)

/p/ ☐   /f/ ☐   /th/ ☐

Do you know why you found some sounds harder than others?

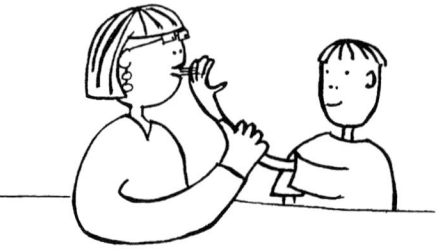

6.10 Tongue tip to alveolar ridge sounds: /t/d/n/r/l/

NAME: DATE:

ACTIVITY   Looking, feeling and doing

First wash your hands.

- Look at the picture of the mouth on Sheet 6.3.
- Find the name 'alveolar ridge'.
- Now open your mouth and put the end of your thumb into your mouth (as though you are going to suck your thumb), put it up onto the rough area just behind your top front teeth (alveolar ridge) and press hard.
- Now take your thumb away. Can you still feel the place where you pressed hard? If not, try again.
- Take your hand mirror, press the alveolar ridge again with your thumb, now lift up your tongue and put the tip of your tongue onto the spot you have just pressed.
- This is where the tongue tip goes to make the consonants /t/d/n/l/r/, so it's a very busy and important place.
- /t/d/ are short sounds. /n/ is a long sound, and with /l/ you can make it a long or a short sound.

Which sounds can you now manage on their own? (tick the box)

	Yes	No	Nearly
Can you make the sound /n/?			
Can you make the sound /l/?			
Can you make the sound /r/?			
Can you make the sound /d/?			
Can you make the sound /t/?			

Lift tongue tip to alveolar ridge (behind upper front teeth)

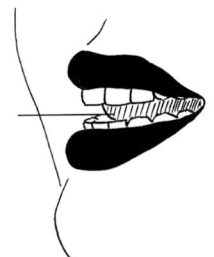

If you can manage some of these sounds you're doing really well. /t/ and /d/ are both short consonants, made in exactly the same place in our mouth. /d/ has a buzz but /t/ is just air.

ACTIVITY   Listening

Get someone to do this with you at home or at school. Ask your helper to say the sounds several times in any order. Listen for any voice buzz, then tick the box for each sound.

	/ppp/	/rrrr/	/ddd/	/ttt/	/bbb/	/nnn/	/lll/
Buzz							
No buzz							

/p/ and /t/ are both sounds with lots of air, so you can feel them on the back of your hand. Feel your voice box to make sure that /p/ and /t/ don't buzz!

6.11 Two other sounds made with tongue tip to alveolar ridge: /s/ and /z/

NAME: DATE:

Look again at column 3 on your sound chart (Sheet 6.4b). Look right at the middle of column 3 for the two consonants /s/ and /z/.

- /s/ is very important because it is used so much in speaking.
- /s/ is often combined with other consonants to make sounds close together, for example the /st/ in stamp, the /sp/ in spoon, the /sk/ in skip, the /sl/ in sleep, the /sm/ in smoke, the /sn/ in snow and the /sw/ in swing.
- /s/ and /z/ are both long sounds, /s/ is the voiceless consonant and /z/ is the voiced one of the pair.
- /s/ is made by putting the tongue tip up to the alveolar ridge and the air streaming out, like down a straw in the middle of the tongue.
- We need to put our tongue on the spot we felt for making /t/ and /d/. Do you remember? If you're not sure, look back at Sheet 6.10. Some people find it more comforable to let their tongue rest down behind their bottom teeth. This is fine if you find that you can make a clear /s/ sound in this way.

ACTIVITY

Teeth together
Smiling lips
Make a hissing sound for /s/
Make a buzzing sound for /z/

Feeling

Look at yourself in a mirror. Open your mouth wide and put the end of your thumb on to the alveolar ridge, and press the spot. Now close your teeth and smile, showing your front teeth together. This is the mouth shape you need for /s/. It is also the mouth shape you need for /z/.

How do you manage these two sounds? (Tick the box)	Yes	No	Nearly
Can you say the sound /s/ on its own?			
Can you say the /z/ sound on its own?			

ACTIVITY   Listening

Ask someone at home or at school to read the words below to you. Tick the box for the voiced (with buzz) or voiceless (air) sound.

	zoo	soap	razor	house	dozen	sink	buzz	seat	face
Buzz									
No buzz									

6.12 Another air sound: /sh/

NAME: DATE:

There's a sound some people use quite a lot, as a reminder to keep quiet. Perhaps the baby is asleep, or someone is ill, or someone is trying to be heard, so we say /sh/. People usually put a finger in front of their lips, and push their lips towards their finger. Perhaps your teacher says it to remind the class to be quiet.

ACTIVITY   **Feeling and doing**

Get someone at home or at school to do this with you. Ask your helper to make the /sh/ sound on your finger. Can you feel that the air is quite warm? Now get your helper to make /f/ on your finger. This time, the air is quite cool. Get your helper to do both sounds several times. If you feel that you can make the sounds yourself (no voice buzz), then you make them on your helper's finger.

If you look on the sound chart (Sheet 6.4b), you'll see that there's another sound in Column 4 (/ʒ/). You know that /sh/ is an air-only sound, but it does have a voiced sound pair (just as /s/ and /z/ are a pair). Its pair has a voice buzz and it comes in words like measure and treasure. There isn't a special letter for writing the sound, but there is a symbol letter to show how it sounds. This is /ʒ/.

The /sh/ sound is nearly always written with the two letters 's' and 'h', and we hear it in words such as **sh**oe, wa**sh**ing, mu**sh**y and fi**sh**. You can probably think of a lot more.

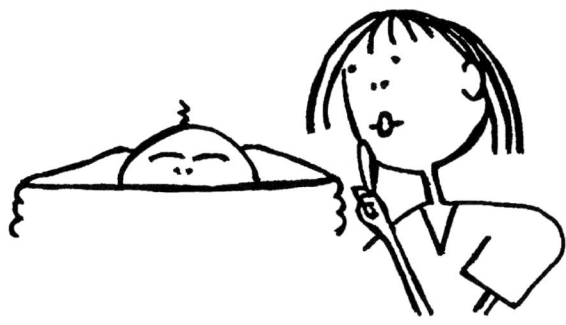

ACTIVITY   **Thinking and writing**

Write a list of words with the /sh/ sound in them:

-
-
-
-
-

When one sound is written with two letters, it is called a digraph – you may already know this word. 'sh' is a digraph, and others are 'ch' and 'th' and 'ph' (which is the /f/ sound in words like 'photo'). There are a few words where /sh/ is written with an 's' like in 'sugar'. Isn't English spelling complicated!

6.13 More sounds with lip rounding: /ch/ and /j/

NAME: DATE:

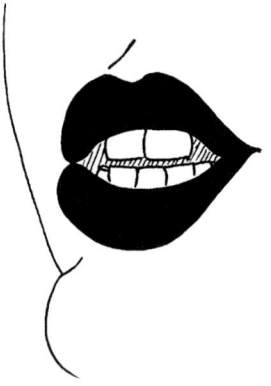

Bring lips forward
Push out air to make a
short sound

/sh/ is an easy sound to see when someone is speaking, because the lips come forward. As you know, this is a long sound, so we can lengthen it out and really see the lips pushing forward – try it, looking in the mirror.

There are two other sounds that we can see with lips pushing forward: the pair of sounds /ch/ and /j/.

- /ch/ is the voiceless air sound. It is a short sound, so the lips push forward and then spring back. It is in words such as **ch**air, wat**ch** and pin**ch**ing.
- /j/ is made with the same movement of the lips, but it also has the voice buzz. It is in words such as **j**am, ba**dg**e and e**dg**ing – notice that it has some different spellings.
- /ch/ is the voiceless air consonant and /j/ is the voiced buzzing consonant. It is more difficult to hear the voice in a short sound.
- /ch/ and /j/ are both short sounds.

ACTIVITY   Listening and doing

Ask someone at home or at school to do this with you Get your helper to say /**ch**/ and /j/ sounds in any order. Use the boxes below to tick the air sound or voice sound.

	/ch/	/j/
Air sound		
Voice buzz		

Now feel the /**ch**/ on the back of your hand. Can you feel the burst of cool air? Then put your fingers on your helper's voice box and ask them to say /j/. Can you feel the buzz on your fingers in this sound? Which of these sounds can you manage? (tick the box)

	Yes	No	Nearly
Can you make the sound /**sh**/ on its own?			
Can you make the /**ch**/ sound on its own?			
Can you make the /j/ sound on its own?			

These sounds are all quite difficult to get exactly right, so if you can manage or nearly manage any of them, you're doing really well.

6.14 A pair of sounds at the back of the mouth: /k/ and /g/

NAME: DATE:

For the vowel 'ah' we need to open our mouth really wide. When someone is speaking at a good speed it is difficult to see inside their mouth. /k/ and /g/ are two sounds where we need to open our mouth well and get our tongue to lift up at the back to meet the soft palate.

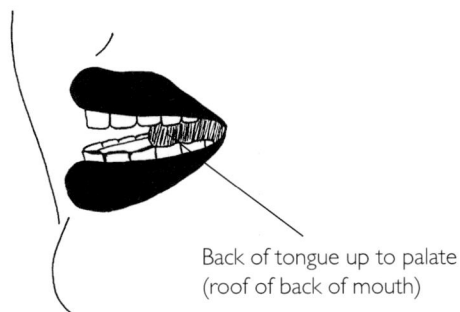

Back of tongue up to palate
(roof of back of mouth)

ACTIVITY   **Looking and listening**

Ask someone at home or at school to do this with you. Both of you should have a look at the picture of the mouth on Sheet 6.3. Check that you know where the soft palate is.

- Look in your hand mirror, or a large mirror if you have one big enough for both of you to see. Both of you open your mouth wide to say 'ah' – can you see right back as far as the end of your soft palate (uvula)?
- Now ask your helper to say these sounds as you look into their mouth: **k k k   g g g**
- Can you see how for both sounds the front of the tongue stays down behind the lower teeth, and the whole of the middle of the tongue lifts up to reach the hard palate? When this happens the back of the palate and uvula is hidden.
- Some people may not have a uvula, or it may be uneven or very short.
- As /k/ and /g/ are both short sounds, the back of the tongue kicks up and then comes down really quickly.
- You have probably spotted the difference between /k/ and /g/. The /k/ consonant is the voiceless air sound and the /g/ is the voiced sound.

ACTIVITY   Can you manage to make these sounds? (Tick one of the boxes)

	Yes	No	Nearly
Can you make the /k/ sound on its own?			
Can you make the /g/ sound on its own?			

Some people find it quite difficult to get the back of their tongue up to their soft palate/uvula. Is this difficult for you? If so, take your hand mirror and look at your open mouth – think about moving your tongue up and back, keeping the tip of your tongue behind your lower front teeth. Say 'ah' several times, be sure the tongue tip stays down.

Now try 'ahk' 'ahk' 'ahk', very slowly.

6.15a A quiz about making speech sounds

NAME: DATE:

Here are some questions about the last sheets you have been working on. Have a go and see how you get on. Go right through to the end, and then if you're not sure of the answer look back to find the sheet with the information you need.

1. Can you list some ways in which we use speech?

2. Which parts of the body do we use for speaking?

3. Do you know another name for the voice box?

4. How many places in the mouth can you name which we use to make speech sounds?

5. Is the tongue a fixed or a moving part?

6. Are the teeth fixed or moving parts?

7. Name the two parts of the mouth used to make the sound /f/.

8. Name the two parts of the mouth used to make the sound /th/.

9. Name two sounds that are made in the same place in the mouth.

10. Are all vowel sounds voiced? (tick one)   Yes   No

6.15b A quiz about making speech sounds (continued)

NAME: DATE:

11. Name two sounds that are just air.

12. Where does the tongue tip have to tap to say /t/ and /d/?

13. If /t/ and /d/ are both made at the same place in the mouth, what is the difference between them?

14. How many sounds can you think of that have lip rounding?

15. Name two long sounds.

16. When we say /bbbb/ is there a voice buzz? (tick one) Yes   No

17. What is the difference between /p/ and /b/?

18. Can you name one difference between /f/ and /p/?

19. Which two sounds do we make right at the back of the mouth?

20. What other sounds can you make that you don't use for speech?

21. Do you have any special sounds not used in speaking English? (tick one) Yes   No

22. Can you write down any non-English sounds?

section 7

What to do if your message is not understood

NAME: DATE:

The important thing about talking is to get your message across to the other person or people whom you are with. However clearly we speak (even when we use our very best speech), there are times when we feel people either don't understand us, or aren't listening. Sometimes we feel it's our fault, sometimes we blame the other person, or maybe we just give up. It depends how important it is to us. If we decide to say something, then it's worth saying!

- When we talk there is usually someone, or several people, who we hope are listening.
- In any speaking situation, there are listeners and talkers. So in any speaking situation, you might be the listener, the talker or both.

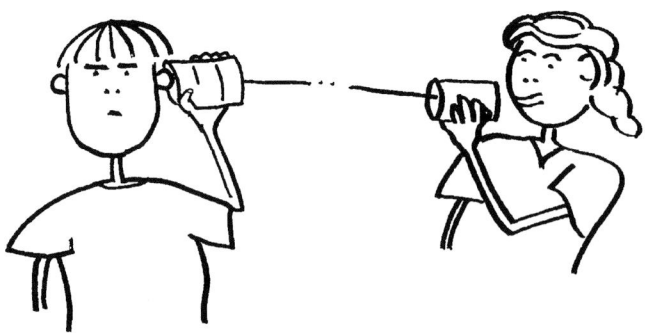

ACTIVITY   Can you think of a situation when you are:

- only a listener?
- only a talker?
- both listener and talker?

Write your ideas here, or discuss them with your helper.

NAME: DATE:

When we talk with someone, it's usually a two-way activity. Even if we are expected to be listening, there are things we can do to make the listening easier.

ACTIVITY   Watch your favourite TV programme – soaps are good for this activity. When people are talking to each other, what do they do to help 'get the message across'? This could be something to discuss with your helper, or someone in your family or a friend. Remember, it takes a talker and a listener to communicate, so:

- What does the talker do?

- What does the listener do?

We'll think more about this later, so don't worry if you can't think of many ideas. There are things you can do to help the talking 'flow' whether you are talking or listening.

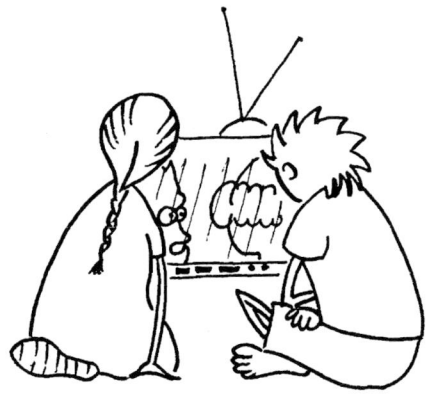

7.3 Listening

NAME: DATE:

You may have talked about listening at school or with your speech and language therapist. Sometimes, when we are listening, we are so busy thinking about what to say next that we find it hard to listen, especially if we are meeting someone for the first time, or want to make a good impression. We all know what it feels like to be 'tongue-tied'! Try your relaxation techniques (Sheets 2.3a and 2.3b)

ACTIVITY   Here are some things to think about, if you are the listener:
- Look at the other person.
- Look interested.
- If you don't hear, or don't understand, let them know. Say: 'I'm sorry, I didn't quite hear that', or, 'Could you say that again, please?'
- If the talker has used a word you didn't understand, ask what it means. It is very difficult to listen to someone if you don't understand what they are saying! We tend to 'switch off'.

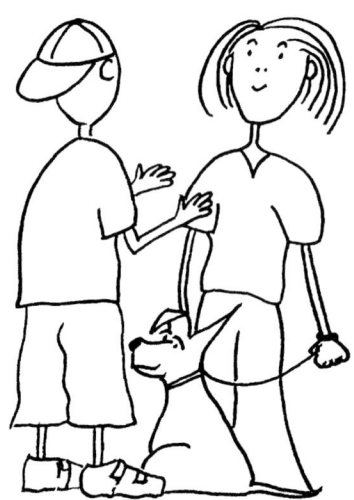

ACTIVITY   Remember what it is like to be the talker. When you are talking, how do you like the listener to behave? Write your ideas here. Can you add anything to the list above?

Thinking about this will make you a better listener, but of course you need to put your ideas into practice!

7.4 Listening: What can go wrong?

NAME: DATE:

When you have been a listener, for example, when your teacher is speaking to the whole class, and has asked you to listen, what can happen to make it difficult for you to listen? Here are some ideas – tick those that have happened to you:

- You are thinking about something else.
- The speaker is not looking at you (facing the board, perhaps).
- Someone near you is talking or making another noise.
- The teacher is talking too quietly.
- The teacher is talking too quickly.
- You don't understand the words used.
- The speaker says too much at one time, so you cannot follow the ideas.
- It's boring, you're not interested in the subject.
- There is another noise in the room (such as a heater or a computer) or even a noise outside (such as an aeroplane).

Can you think of any more?

These can apply to any listening situation. Think what you could do to help your listening. Talking and listening go together, so what helps us listen can also be what helps the talking flow.

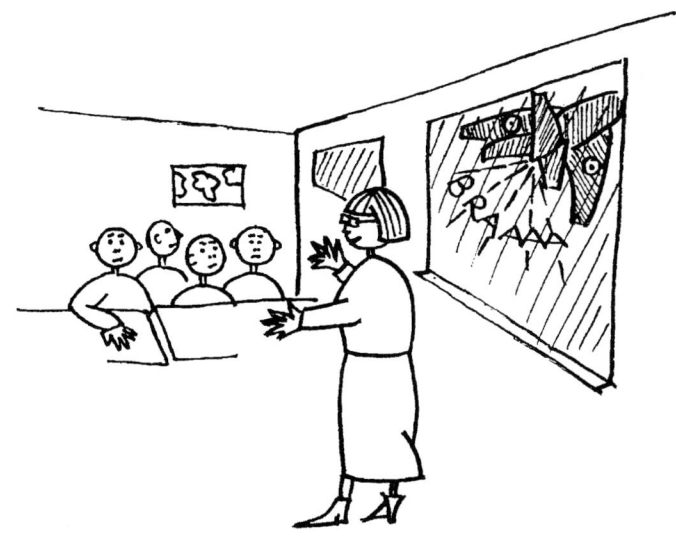

7.5 Practise your listening

NAME: DATE:

To be a good LISTENER, there are some things we need to remember:

- Pay attention.
- Look at the talker – if you haven't heard or understood, you may get clues from their body, hands or face. More about this later.
- Indicate that you are interested, and that you have understood, perhaps by smiling or nodding, or by making a comment about what the other person is talking about. For example, if they are talking about a favourite record, you could say whether it is good to dance to.
- Try not to interrupt too much! (that's hard for everyone)
- Ask, if you haven't understood or heard.

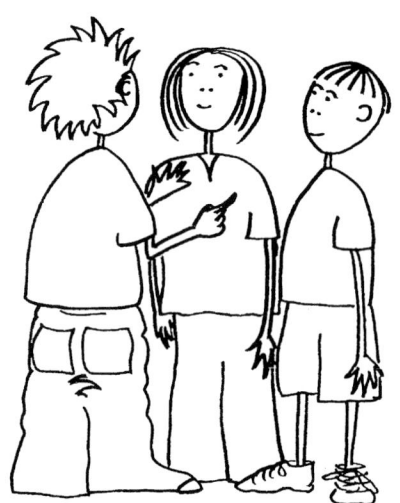

ACTIVITY   Practise these skills in some of the speaking situations in Section 8 (Making the best use of your voice and speech). Then use the Evaluation Sheets to think about how it went (Sheets 8.14 and 8.15).

7.6 Talking

NAME: DATE:

Here are some things to think about when you are the TALKER:

- Think about the listener.
- Don't say too much in one go. It's hard to listen for a long time, so take turns to talk and listen.
- Look at your listeners in a friendly way. Smile!
- Speak up – not too quietly, or too loudly.
- Speak out – not too quickly.
- Hold your head up.
- Use your best speech (all the things that help others to understand you, like looking up and opening your mouth).
- Use your face, hands and body to help get your message across.

Remember to make the most of what you CAN do.

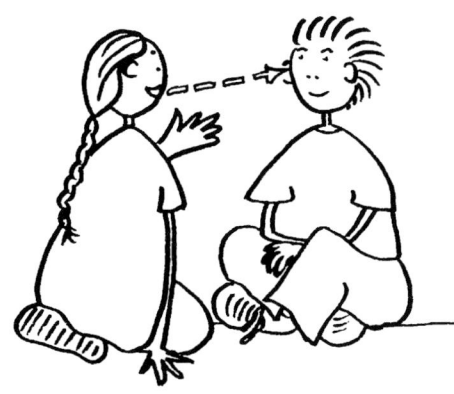

ACTIVITY Practise these skills in some of the speaking situations in Section 8 (Making the best use of your voice and speech). Then use the evaluation sheets to think about how it went (Sheets 8.14 and 8.15)

7.7 Not only words I: Non-verbal communication

NAME: DATE:

It isn't only the words we use, or the way we say them, that matters.

ACTIVITY Watch your favourite video or soap on television again. Turn the sound down for a few minutes (you can do this with something you have recorded earlier, if you don't want to miss the programme).

Can you guess what the people are talking about? Can you tell how they feel? Write your ideas here:

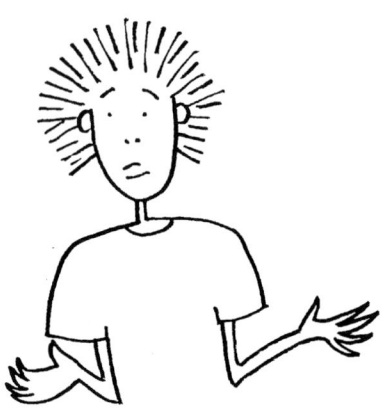

ACTIVITY You can help to get your message across by using your face, your arms and hands or your body position. You probably do this already, without even noticing. If you get the chance, it can be interesting to watch yourself on a video to see what you do when you are talking. Turn the sound down and watch. Not many of us enjoy the experience, but it can be useful!

There are more activities to try on the next sheet (Sheet 7.8).

7.8 Not only words 2: More activities to try

NAME: DATE:

Here are some more activities to try.

ACTIVITY   Try to explain how to do something without talking. For example, show someone how to make a cup of tea or how to get to your school from your house. Remember, no talking!

ACTIVITY   Now repeat the activity above, using only words. Remember, no hands! Sit on them if it helps. Which activity did you find easier? Some people use their hands more than others. Some people are better with words. Ask the person listening which was easier to follow.

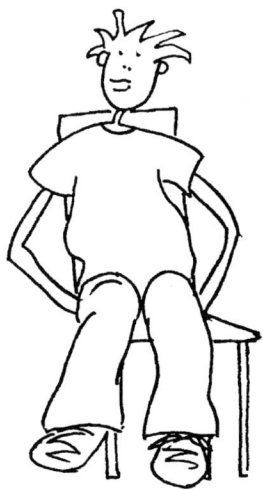

7.9 Talking: What can go wrong?

NAME: DATE:

We have talked about being a listener and a talker. When you are listening, we said how important it is to let the other person know when you haven't heard or understood.

This will happen when you are the talker too! The person who is listening to you is likely to ask you to say something again, or explain it. If you have speech difficulties, you may think they haven't understood you because of the way you talk. This may be the case, but there are lots of other reasons why someone may ask you to repeat something! What could they be? Any ideas?

ACTIVITY Look back at the 'Listening' sheets for ideas (Sheets 7.1–7.5), and write them here:

ACTIVITY Make a list of reasons why someone may ask you to repeat something.

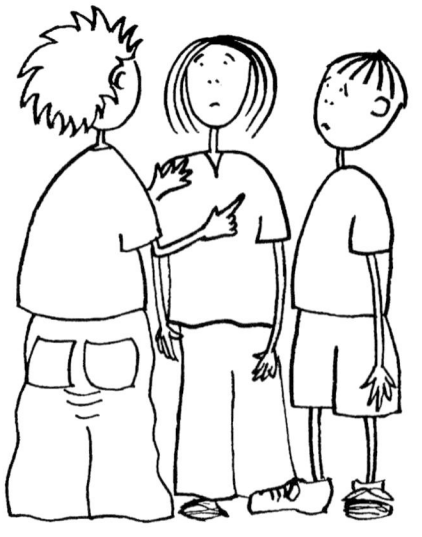

NAME: DATE:

ACTIVITY Here are some reasons why you might be asked to say something again:

- The person may not have been listening properly.
- There may be some background noise.
- They may not have understood the words, or may not be used to the way you talk.
- They may have found it difficult to remember, if you have said a lot!

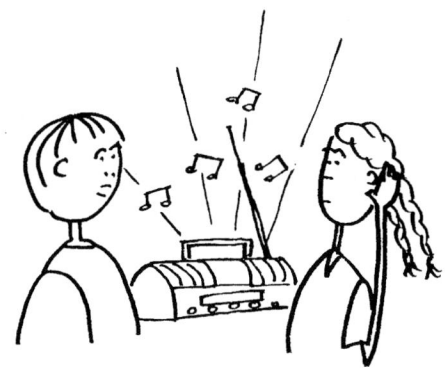

So, before you say it again:

- Make sure the place where you are isn't too noisy. Move to a quieter spot if possible.
- Say it in a different way if you think the words were too difficult.
- Say it a bit at a time, and check the other person has understood each part before you continue.
- If they weren't listening, make sure they are this time!
- And remember: USE YOUR BEST SPEECH!

If someone doesn't understand you, what might they do? Here are some ideas, you may think of others.

- Ignore you.
- Walk away.
- Ask you to say it again, politely.
- Say 'What?'
- Talk to someone else.

Which would you find the most helpful?

7.11 Getting the message across: Quiz

NAME: DATE:

So, you know a lot about talking and listening, and what you can do to help. Remember it takes listeners and talkers to make a conversation flow. Can you answer these questions?

- What is the best thing you can do if it is too noisy to listen easily?

- How do you know if someone has understood you?

- What helps 'get your message across' apart from the words?

- Write down three things that can make listening difficult:

  1.

  What can you do to help?

  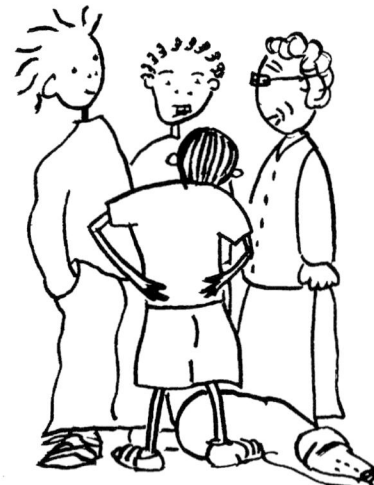

  2.

  What can you do to help?

  3.

  What can you do to help?

- Think of three ways to help 'get your message across' – this time think about how you talk:

7.12 Evaluation sheet – getting the message across: How did it go?

NAME: DATE:

ACTIVITY Speaking situation
Think of the last time you were with someone you hadn't spoken to before, and think about how you got on.

- Describe the situation (eg was the other person older or younger than you, where were you, what were you doing?)

- Were you the talker / listener / both (circle one)

- How did it go? very well / OK/ not very well
  (circle one)

Give yourself a mark out of 10 for:

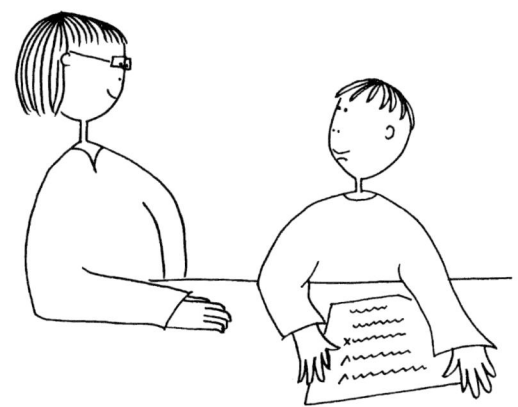

- Looking at the other person   /10

- Looking friendly or interested   /10

- Not interrupting   /10

- Using your best speech   /10

Were you asked to say anything again? (circle one) Yes / No
If the answer is yes, why do you think that was?

Did you have to ask the other person to repeat anything? If yes, why?

section 8

Making the best use of your voice and speech

8.1 Whispering your way to clear gentle speech

NAME: DATE:

Although we don't often need to speak in a whisper, you may find it a good way to help you to make very clear sounds in your mouth, because we don't need to use the voice buzz at all.

ACTIVITY   **Relaxing**

First we need to relax our shoulders and necks. There are some ideas about relaxation in Section 2. If someone at home has some nice smelling face or body cream, it helps to relax if you rub cream around your throat and neck. As you do this you can tell your voice box to go to sleep – because it can stay quiet.

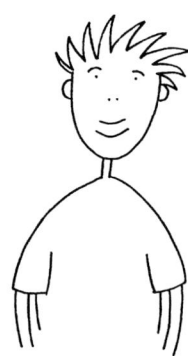

Look back to the sheets on relaxation (Sheets 2.1–2.3b), and go over the exercises that you found especially helpful.

You already know about the voice box in your throat, and that its proper name is larynx. Here is a picture of a larynx. It looks rather funny, a bit like a cowboy with no eyes.

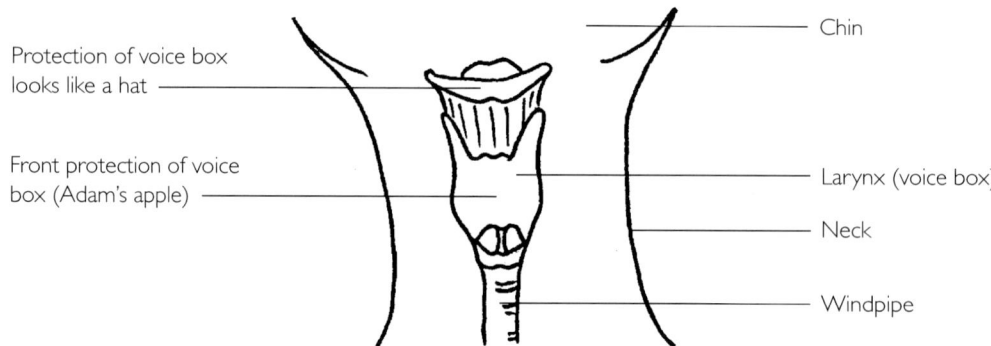

Protection of voice box looks like a hat

Front protection of voice box (Adam's apple)

Chin

Larynx (voice box)

Neck

Windpipe

8.2 Your larynx doesn't have to do all the work

NAME: DATE:

ACTIVITY Larynx man
While the larynx man is asleep, we can whisper – remember, no voice buzz!

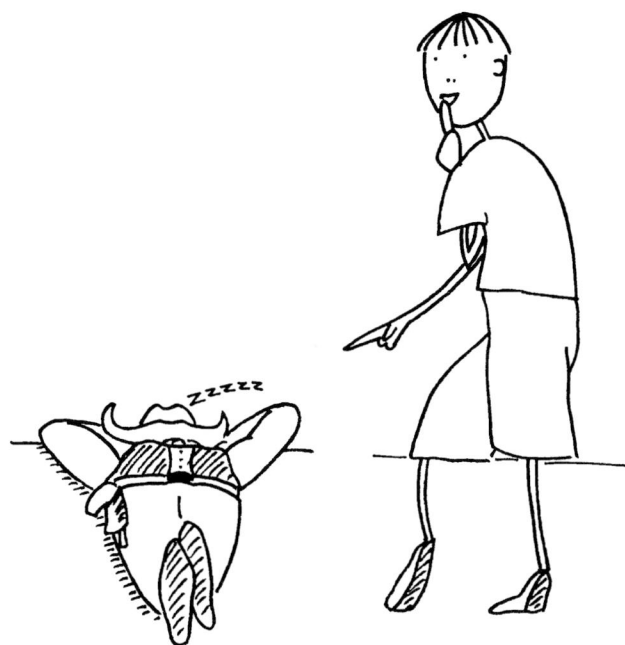

ACTIVITY Can you whisper a bit more? Here are some good whispery words. See if you can say them with a clear gentle whisper. Do not force any of the sounds. Each time you whisper a word, put your fingers on your larynx to make sure there isn't any voice buzz

whisper	touching	chocolate	puppy	shoe shop
spitting	sausages	pussy cat	paper	shopping
stamps	cutting	pushing	cushion	

Ask someone to help you to think of some more words.

8.3 Easy does it: Gentle ways to speak

NAME: DATE:

If we find it difficult to make some sounds clearly with our lips or tongue, like /p/b/t/d/k/g/, we may make them in our voice box instead. As you already know /b/d/g/ are all sounds that have the voice buzz (voiced sounds), so that will be not too bad. But /p/t/k/ are voiceless consonants — so if we make a voice buzz with them that's very confusing for the listener and we also make a really hard ∗∗∗∗∗∗∗∗ BANG ∗∗∗∗∗∗∗∗ with those precious vocal folds in our voice box.

ACTIVITY **Feeling**

It may be quite a while since you checked your sound making. You may have been working on some new sounds. Let's see how you're getting on with making the short voiceless consonants. Put your fingers on your voice box, as you learned to do on sheet 5.1. Now say the following sounds very gently, and tick whether you feel any buzz or not.

	p p p	t t t	k k k
Buzz			
No buzz			

Remember, there should **not** be any voice buzz on your finger tips.

- If you can do all three sounds with no buzz that's marvellous.
- If you do two with no voice buzz, then you're coming along well. If you do just one of the consonants without a buzz then you've made a good start.
- If you still find it very hard to keep out the voice buzz, then we need to try to find out why.

Perhaps you're trying too hard — go very gently. Sometimes if we feel tense, tight and not relaxed, our voice bands (vocal folds) come too close together and may bang or buzz by mistake.

Go over some of the activities on relaxation (Sheets 2.1–2.3b). Now that you're feeling really floppy and calm, and not trying too hard, make the three sounds again (/p/t/k/). Remember to put your fingers on your voice box. Perhaps one of the sounds is easier than the others. Make the sounds again and then fill in these boxes with a tick:

Which sound is the easiest?   /**p**/ ☐   /**t**/ ☐   /**k**/ ☐
Which sound is the hardest?   /**p**/ ☐   /**t**/ ☐   /**k**/ ☐

ACTIVITY Here are two pictures of the voice bands vibrating. Which picture do you think would make your voice hurt?

8.4 Saying the voiced vowel sounds gently

NAME: DATE:

You already know that some sounds are made with the voice bands buzzing, some of the consonants and all the vowels. When a word starts with a vowel we need to be careful that we don't make it like an explosion. That really bangs the voice bands together and hurts them.

ACTIVITY **Saying vowels gently**

A good way to learn to go gently with vowels is by saying another word that is almost the same, but starts with /h/, which is a very gentle air sound. When we make a /h/ consonant the voice bands come quite close together, but don't touch, so the air passing through them makes a long sighing kind of sound – /hhhhhhhhhhh/. Say it now, and feel the warm air on the back of your hand. We also make this sound when we sigh.

Now try to say some words beginning with /h/. Make sure that you are very relaxed, so that the /h/ comes out very smoothly and gently.

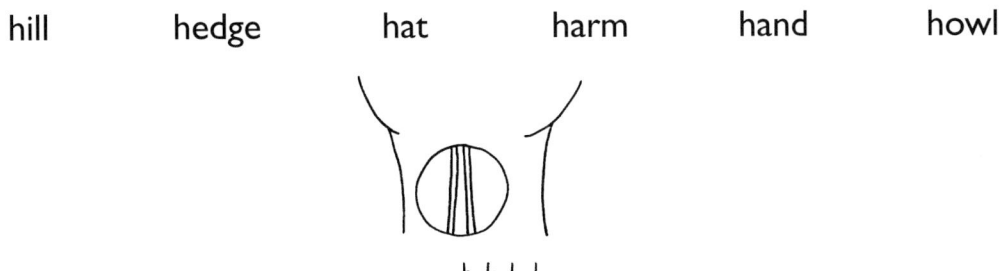

| hill | hedge | hat | harm | hand | howl |

h h h h

You may have noticed that if you take the /h/ off the front of the word, you have a new word with a different meaning. Now try the matching word pairs below. Say the first word followed by the second. Think about the /h/ before the word starting with a vowel, but don't sound it aloud. Listen to yourself carefully. Put a tick in the box if you think you said the vowel gently, and a cross if you think it was too much of a bang. If you're not sure how you're getting on, ask someone to listen to you. Here are the matching pairs:

	Matching pairs of word					
	hill ill	harm arm	hedge edge	hand and	hat at	howl owl
Gently						
Banged						

Have you still got someone helping you? Together perhaps you can find some more word pairs and try saying them. Here are a few more examples. Can you work out the second word? Fill in the second word and then practice it. Sometimes the spelling may change a bit.

hair _____   Hannah _____   had _____

Now make your own list. Take a new sheet of paper, or use the other side of this sheet. You may find it takes a while to think of the words.

8.5 Thinking about our best speech

NAME: DATE:

What we mean by 'best' speech is using all the things we've learned about that help people to understand what we want to say. Speaking is hard for some people:

- They may have had an accident that affects the way they speak.
- Their brain might work differently, so this might affect how fluently or clearly they speak.
- They may have difficulty hearing the sounds they say, or the sounds other people say, so they may use different sound patterns to make words when they talk.
- They may have been born with noticeable differences of their lips and/or palate.

These are some of the reasons they may need to work harder at getting other people to understand what they are saying.

ACTIVITY   Try talking with your mouth closed, or your teeth together (like a ventriloquist!)

- What happens?
- Is it easy to understand what you are saying?

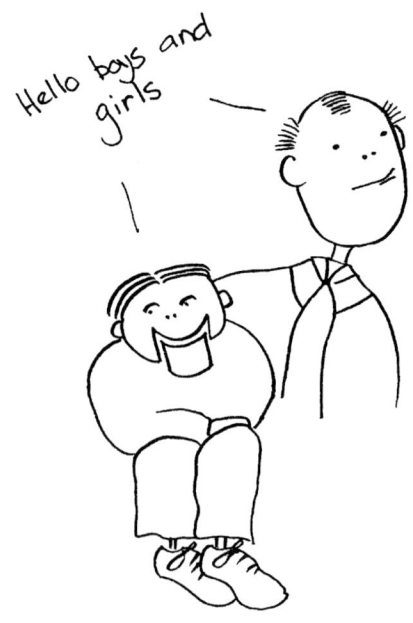

NAME: DATE:

Some people – maybe you are one of them – work for months, maybe years, to improve the way they speak, to make it easier for people to understand them. As well as working on speech sounds, there are lots of other things you can do to help people understand you better. As with most things in life, we need to make the best use of the skills we have. Like all skills, from swimming to drawing a picture, there are days when we feel things went well, and days when we just couldn't do it, no matter how hard we tried!

Sheets 8.9–8.16 will help you think about your best speech, and what you can do to help yourself. And remember – your best speech is just that – yours! It won't be quite like anyone else's, because we are all unique.

Watch your favourite TV programme. Can you find two people who talk in the same way?

ACTIVITY Choose one or two of your favourite characters. Do they speak:

- Slowly or quickly?

- In a high voice or a low voice?

- In a quiet voice or a loud voice?

- With a different accent?

- In a tense or relaxed way?

- Is the way they speak lively and interesting, or flat and boring?

- How much do they open their mouth when they talk?

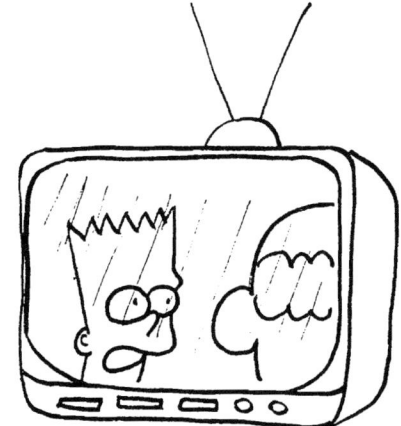

Talk about this with someone. You may have different ideas.

8.7 Flat and wavy talking 1

ACTIVITY
- Can you speak like a robot?! Try to do this now.
- How is this different from the way you usually talk?

Robots sound strange and boring. Real people usually make their words go 'up and down' to sound more interesting. We could call this 'wavy talking', or maybe you could think of your own word to describe it. You could think of the way a robot speaks as 'flat talking'. We also make some words STRONGER than others.

ACTIVITY Look at this sentence: say it like a robot! It sounds strange, doesn't it?

I like strawberry ice cream.

You could say it like this: make your voice go up or down following the arrows

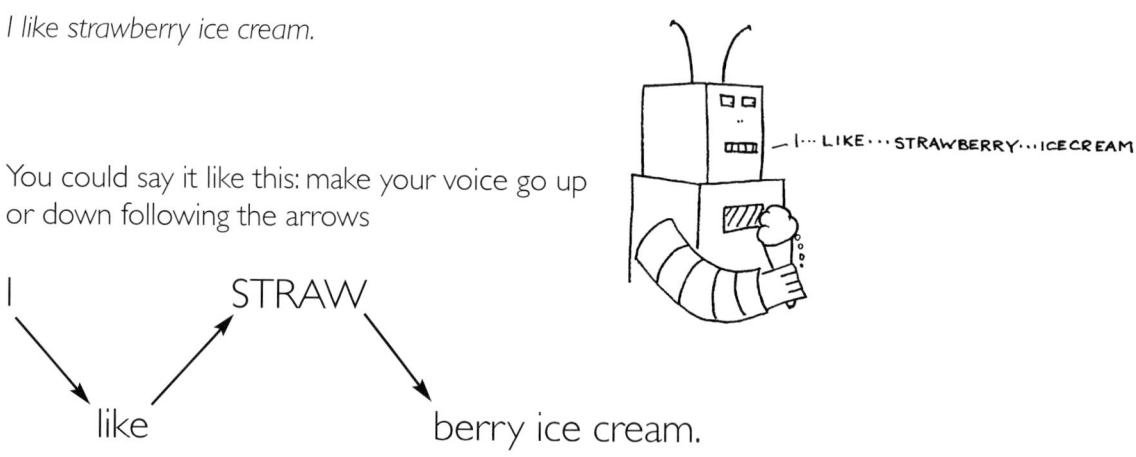

or:

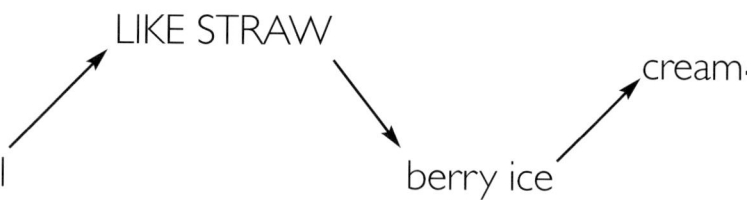

They mean something slightly different, don't they? Talk about this with your helper.

8.8 Flat and wavy talking 2

NAME: DATE:

On Sheet 8.7, the sentences you tried went 'up and down'. Some words, or parts of words (syllables), were stronger than others when you said them. Another way of saying this is that you put STRESS on some words.

ACTIVITY   **Think about 'wavy talking'**
Look at this sentence. How many different ways can you say it? Do this activity with your helper; ask them to do the writing if you like – you do the thinking.

Do you want a packet of crisps?

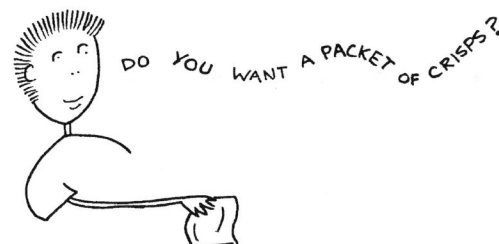

ACTIVITY
- Choose three different sentences you see written on this sheet, and write them down in the space below.
- Take each sentence in turn, underline the words you stressed when you said the sentence aloud.
- Talk with your helper about what each sentence means when you say it in a different way.
- Perhaps you could think of some more sentences you could do this with.

1.

2.

3.

8.9 Using your best speech: Why?

NAME: DATE:

Why do we need to use our best speech when we talk to people? Perhaps we need to think about who we talk to and why? Here are some of the people you probably talk to:

- friends
- family
- teachers
- people in shops

ACTIVITY   Here are some questions to think about:

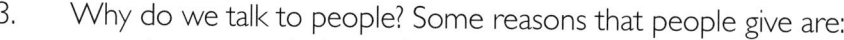

1.   Who else do you talk to? Make your list here:

2.   Are some people easier to talk to than others? Why?

3.   Why do we talk to people? Some reasons that people give are:
- to get peoples' attention
- to tell someone something
- to ask for, or give information
- to tell someone how we feel or what we think
- to be friendly
- to find out about the other person
- to tell people about you
- to ask where to go or what to do
- just because it's fun!

4.   Why do YOU talk to people? Make your list here:

8.10 Using your best speech: When? Where?

NAME: DATE:

ACTIVITY   Think of different situations where you use talking.

Where do you talk to people? At school? At home? With friends? Family? To your class? Reading aloud? On the phone? In shops? On the bus? Add your ideas to the list below, and give each situation a mark out of 10 for how easy or difficult you find it. (1 = hard, 10 = very easy)

- talking to a friend   /10
- talking to a grown-up at home   /10
- talking to brother/sister   /10
- talking to teacher   /10
- talking in a shop   /10
- talking to someone for the first time   /10
- talking on the phone   /10
- talking in front of my class   /10
- talking in a group of friends   /10

-   /10
-   /10
-   /10
-   /10
-   /10
-   /10
-   /10

8.11 What is your best speech?

NAME: DATE:

What do we mean by your 'best speech'? Do you 'mumble'? Sometimes we don't need to speak louder, but just open our mouths more. If our mouths are nearly closed when we talk, it can come out as a 'mumble-jumble'! Most people mumble sometimes. It is really important to speak out so the listener can hear and understand you. Talk about this with your therapist, or a friend or someone in your family.

ACTIVITY   What can you do to be the best talker you can be?

It isn't only about working on speech sounds. Do you need to do any of the things in the following list? (Tick the ones that you think you need to think about.)

- slow down?
- speak up?
- open your mouth more?
- look at the person or people listening to you?
- practise your special sounds more?
- make your talking more 'wavy'?

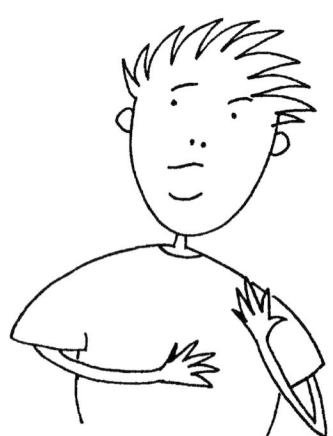

Remember, using your best speech means using your best voice too! See: 'Ways to keep your voice in good shape' on Sheet 5.6, and other activities in that section (How your voice works).

ACTIVITY   What is your best speech? What do you need to do? Write your ideas here:

8.12 Practising your best speech

NAME: DATE:

ACTIVITY   Stand up tall! Choose one of the situations from the list on Sheet 8.10: pretend you are in that situation (for example, in a shop). Decide what you are going to say.

Practise using your best speech
You could do this in front of a mirror (or video yourself), or ask someone friendly to listen to you, or video you. Remember: most people are nervous about speaking to other people for the first time.

How did you do?
Give yourself marks out of 10 for each of the following (1 = hard, 10 = excellent!)

- holding your head up   /10

- opening your mouth as much as you needed to   /10

- speaking as loudly as was needed for the situation   /10

- speaking as slowly as was needed for the situation   /10

- making the sounds as clearly as you could   /10

- speaking in an interesting way ('wavy' talking)   /10

- making eye contact   /10

Do you think you could be understood (tick your answer)?

yes ☐   no ☐   some of the time ☐

This may seem like a lot to think about, but this is just to practise. Like when you learn to swim or ride a bike, there seem to be lots of things to think about at once, but suddenly it all comes together!

8.13 Using your best speech

So now you know what your best speech sounds like. What we feel about the way we talk isn't the same every day — sometimes it feels fine, sometimes it doesn't, depending how we feel on that day. We can only do our best, for that day.

The main thing to think about is whether you manage to 'get your message across', because that's why we talk!

ACTIVITY   Now you have 'pretended' to use your best speech, how about doing the same thing in a real situation? You can use the evaluation Sheets (8.14 and 8.15) to give yourself marks.

Practise as many of the situations as possible. Do this with the help of your speech and language therapist, or another helper.

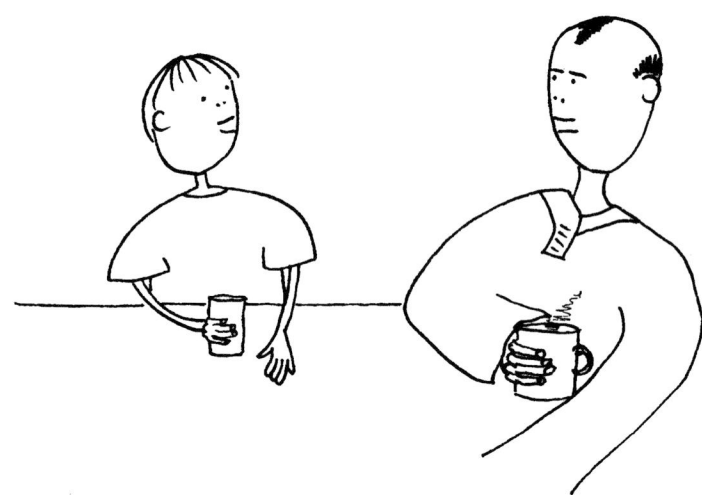

8.14 Evaluation sheet for using your best speech: General impressions

NAME: DATE:

ACTIVITY   **Speaking situation:**
(where you practised your best speech – see Sheet 8.13)

- holding your head up   /10

- making eye contact   /10

- opening your mouth (speaking out)   /10

- looking friendly   /10

- feeling relaxed   /10

- Do you think you could be understood? (tick one box)

  yes ☐   no ☐   some of the time ☐

  How do you know?

- Could you have done anything differently?

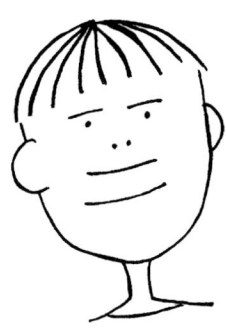 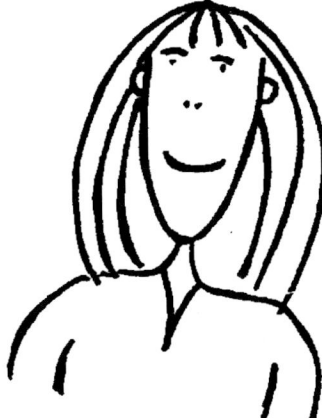

8.15 Evaluation sheet for using your best speech: More detail

NAME: DATE:

ACTIVITY   Speaking situation
(where you practised your best speech – see Sheet 8.13)

- making the sounds as clearly as you could   /10

- speaking as slowly as was needed for the situation   /10

- speaking as loudly/quietly as was needed   /10

- sounding interesting ('wavy' talking)   /10

- feeling/sounding tense or relaxed   /10

- opening your mouth as much as you needed to   /10

- Do you think you could be understood? (tick one box)

  yes ☐   no ☐   some of the time ☐

  How do you know?

- Could you have done anything differently?

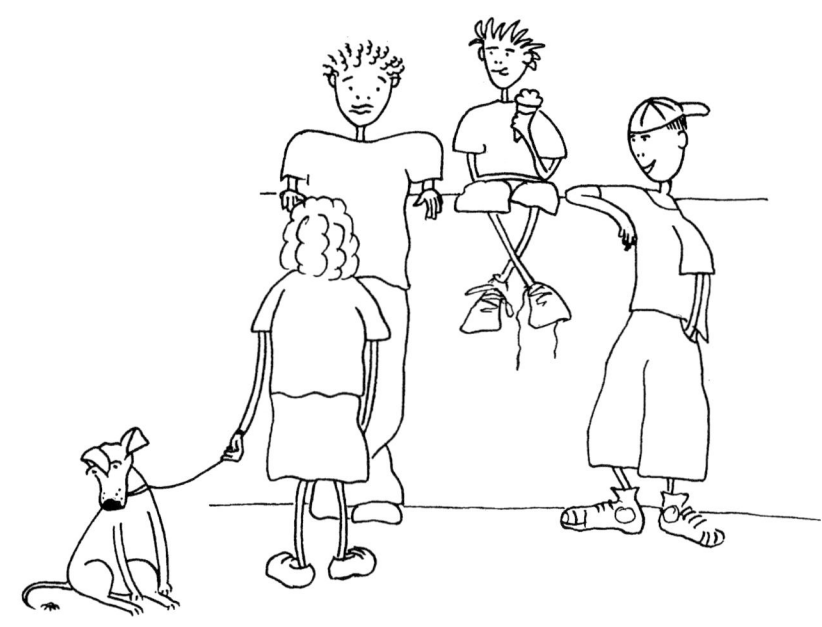

8.16 Using your best speech: A few questions

NAME: DATE:

A few more things to think about: there are no right or wrong answers to the questions below just things you may like to discuss with a friend or helper.

ACTIVITY

• Do you talk in the same way to your teachers/friends/family?

• Are you more likely to use your best speech when you feel comfortable in a situation?

• Which is an easier talking situation? (Please tick **a** or **b** for each example)

Example 1
a. talking with friends about a party
or
b. telling your parents about being in trouble at school

Example 2
a. talking with your family about a planned holiday
or
b. explaining to your teacher why your homework wasn't in on time

• Do you always use your best speech in the easiest situation?

• When are you most likely to want to use your best speech? (please tick)
  – with someone you are meeting for the first time?
  – in a group of friends?
  – when there is a lot of background noise?
  – when you want to attract someone's attention?
  – with someone who knows you well?
  – always?
  – on the telephone?
  – in a shop?

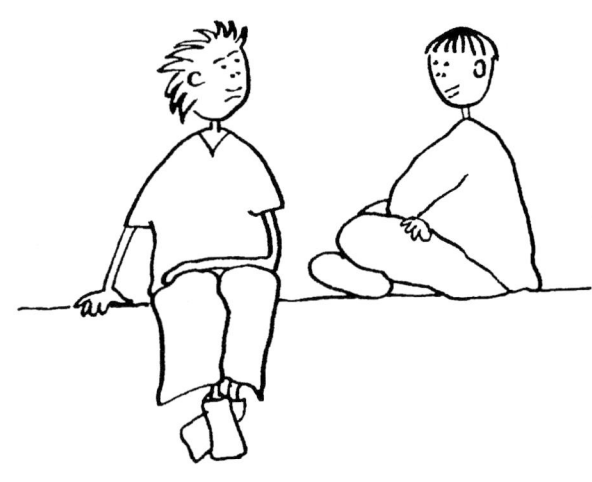